Case Reviews in
Ophthalmology

Case Reviews in Ophthalmology

Second Edition

Neil J. Friedman MD
Adjunct Clinical Associate Professor,
Department of Ophthalmology, Stanford University School of Medicine
Palo Alto, CA, USA
Partner, Mid-Peninsula Ophthalmology Medical Group
Menlo Park, CA, USA

Peter K. Kaiser MD
Chaney Family Endowed Chair for Ophthalmology Research
Professor of Ophthalmology, Cleveland Clinic Lerner College of Medicine
Cole Eye Institute, Cleveland Clinic
Cleveland, OH, USA

Edinburgh   London   New York   Oxford   Philadelphia   St Louis   Sydney   Toronto   2018

Notices

Knowledge and best practice in this field are constantly changing. As new research and experience broaden our understanding, changes in research methods, professional practices, or medical treatment may become necessary.

Practitioners and researchers must always rely on their own experience and knowledge in evaluating and using any information, methods, compounds, or experiments described herein. In using such information or methods they should be mindful of their own safety and the safety of others, including parties for whom they have a professional responsibility.

With respect to any drug or pharmaceutical products identified, readers are advised to check the most current information provided (i) on procedures featured or (ii) by the manufacturer of each product to be administered, to verify the recommended dose or formula, the method and duration of administration, and contraindications. It is the responsibility of practitioners, relying on their own experience and knowledge of their patients, to make diagnoses, to determine dosages and the best treatment for each individual patient, and to take all appropriate safety precautions.

To the fullest extent of the law, neither the Publisher nor the authors, contributors, or editors, assume any liability for any injury and/or damage to persons or property as a matter of products liability, negligence or otherwise, or from any use or operation of any methods, products, instructions, or ideas contained in the material herein.

ISBN: 978-0-323-39059-0
eISBN: 978-0-323-39061-3

Printed in China
Last digit is the print number: 9 8 7 6 5 4 3 2 1

Content Strategist: Russell Gabbedy
Content Development Specialist: Nani Clansey
Content Coordinator: Joshua Mearns
Project Manager: Srividhya Vidhyashankar
Design: Miles Hitchen
Illustration Manager: Amy Faith Heyden
Marketing Manager: Melissa Fogarty

Contents

Preface   vii

Acknowledgments   viii

1. OPTICS/REFRACTION   1

2. NEURO-OPHTHALMOLOGY/ORBIT   47

3. PEDIATRIC OPHTHALMOLOGY/STRABISMUS   95

4. EXTERNAL DISEASE/ADNEXA   149

5. ANTERIOR SEGMENT   201

6. POSTERIOR SEGMENT   251

Index   313

Index of Cases   323

Preface

It has been gratifying to witness the success of *Case Reviews in Ophthalmology*, and we are delighted to present the second edition of this book. The new edition follows the same familiar case-based format with accompanying answers, but we have expanded the contents by adding 30 new cases. Our goal is to present additional topics that are important and relevant to clinicians. We carefully selected the new material to complement the existing cases and to further aid in learning and studying core information that we all must know.

We hope you continue to find this case method of learning helpful for understanding clinical problems as well as preparing for exams.

Neil J. Friedman MD
Peter K. Kaiser MD

Acknowledgments

The updated edition of this book has been a group effort, and we are grateful to all of our colleagues, friends and family who have helped us along the way.

We continue to be blessed to work with a superb team at Elsevier: thank you Russell Gabbedy, Nani Clansey, Srividhya Vidhyashankar, and your incredible staff.

Most importantly, we must thank our families: Mae, Jake, Dawn, Peter (PJ), and Stephanie, who continue to support our book writing habit.

Neil J. Friedman MD
Peter K. Kaiser MD

A 48-year-old woman with myopia complains of progressive deterioration in distance and near vision in both eyes for the past 2 years. She can improve her vision by sliding her glasses down her nose. Her past medical history is significant for diabetes for 10 years, for which she takes glyburide. She reports blood sugar levels usually between 120 and 140 mg/dL and a recent hemoglobin A1c of 6.8%.

1. What is the differential diagnosis?
2. What other history would you like to know?
3. What would your exam entail?

Additional information: her current glasses are −5.00 D with an add of +1.25 D OU, her manifest refraction is −4.25 D OD and −4.50 D OS with +1.50 D add OU. The crystalline lenses are clear OU and there is no diabetic retinopathy. Cycloplegic refraction reveals −4.25 D OU.

4. What is your diagnosis and treatment plan?

1. Decreased myopia and increased presbyopia. The change in refractive error may be due to overcorrection in her current distance spectacle prescription, cataracts, diabetic macular edema, or medications (ie, chloroquine, phenothiazines, antihistamines, benzodiazepines).

2. How old is her current prescription and what type of glasses are they? Does she have glare/halo/starburst from lights? Has the diabetes ever affected her retina and if so did she ever have any retinal treatment? Is she taking any other medications?

3. Measure her current glass prescription, perform a manifest refraction, and then a complete eye exam with attention to the crystalline lens for cataract and retina for diabetic macular edema.

4. Myopia/presbyopia with overminused glasses. A new glasses prescription should be given using the power from her manifest refraction. She should continue good blood sugar control and return for annual eye exams.

A 50-year-old man with low myopia is noticing more difficulty reading with his distance glasses. He usually takes his glasses off to read but says this is becoming a hassle, and therefore he wants a new pair of glasses.

1. What is the problem?
2. What are his options?
3. What are the two prismatic effects that occur with bifocals?
4. Discuss the pros and cons of different bifocal designs.

1. Presbyopia.

2. The glasses options are progressive, bifocal, or single vision lenses. Glasses for the computer can be single vision, trifocal, or computer bifocals.

3. Image jump and image displacement.

   Image jump is related to the position of the optical center of the add segment. It is produced by the sudden prismatic power at the top of the bifocal segment (it is not influenced by the type of underlying lens). As the patient's line of sight crosses from the optical center of the distance lens to the bifocal segment, the image position suddenly shifts up owing to the base-down (BD) prismatic effect of the bifocal segment.

   Image displacement is due to the total prismatic power of the lens and bifocal segment. It is minimized when the prismatic effect of the bifocal segment and distance lens are in opposite directions.

   Image jump is more bothersome than image displacement, so the segment type should be chosen to minimize image jump.

4. The advantage of progressive lenses is the blended segment without a visible line and there is no image jump; however, there is usually an adaptation period, especially for patients who have previously worn lined bifocals.

   Bifocal lenses have a visible line and there are different types of segment styles – round-top, flat-top, and executive. Round-top segments produce the most image jump, and they cause more image displacement in myopes than in hyperopes. Flat-top segments minimize image jump, and image displacement is less in a myope than a hyperope. Executive bifocals have a larger area dedicated to near vision, and there is no image jump because the optical centers are at the top of the segment.

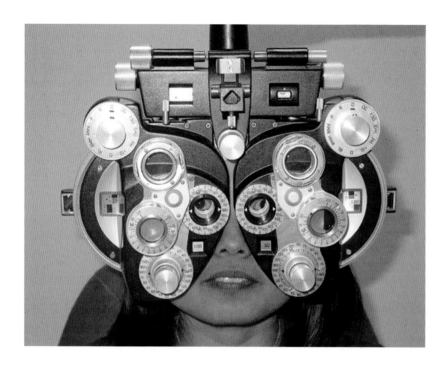

A 46-year-old woman complains of trouble with near vision. Her current glasses are 4 years old and she says her eyes feel strained when she reads. She wants to get a new prescription for glasses.

1. What is the technique for subjective manifest refraction?
2. How would you determine her add power?

1. Starting with her current prescription in either a trial lens or phoropter, the distance vision is checked monocularly and the sphere is adjusted first as she is asked to read progressively smaller lines on the acuity chart. The axis of any cylinder is then refined with a Jackson cross cylinder. The vision must be at least 20/40 to use the 0.25 cross cylinder. Once the correct axis is determined, the amount of cylinder is then determined in a similar fashion with the cross cylinder. The sphere is then rechecked until the best acuity is achieved. Finally, three methods can be used to perform binocular balance to equally control accommodation in both eyes during distance refraction: prism dissociation (3 prism diopters [PD] BU over one eye and 3 PD BD over the other with a Risley prism), balanced fogging (fog both eyes and alternate cover until equally fogged), or duochrome test (red–green balance both eyes).

2. To determine the bifocal add, measure accommodation monocularly then binocularly. A Prince rule (reading card with a ruler calibrated in centimeters and diopters to measure amplitude of accommodation) can be used with the phoropter to determine the necessary accommodative requirement for various near vision tasks. Half of the patient's measured accommodative amplitude should be held in reserve to prevent asthenopia.

   For example, if the patient desires to read at 40 cm (2.5 D), the Prince rule measures 2.0 D of amplitude (1.0 D is available to patient to prevent asthenopic symptoms), then the add power is 1.5 D (the difference between accommodation [1.0 D] and the total amount of accommodation required to read [2.5 D]). With the calculated add in front of the distance correction, measure the accommodative range (near point to far point of accommodation). If the range is too close, then reduce the add in steps of 0.25 D until the correct range is found.

A 31-year-old woman with a refractive error of −2.50 D in both eyes is interested in refractive surgery. She has become contact lens intolerant and glasses interfere with her sports activities and lifestyle.

1. What would you tell her about surgical correction of her myopia?
2. What are the complications of LASIK (laser-assisted in situ keratomileusis)?

Additional information: this patient undergoes LASIK. The day after surgery she is very happy with her 20/20 vision. On exam her left eye has the finding seen in the photo.

3. What is the diagnosis and what would you do?

1. There are a number of surgical options for correcting low myopia. The most common is excisional (laser vision correction [surface ablation, LASIK]). Other techniques include incisional (radial keratotomy) and additive (implants [Intacs]). The indications, risks, benefits, alternatives, and complications of surgery should be discussed as well as the advantages and disadvantages of each of the procedures. She should also be told about what to expect during the preoperative and postoperative periods.

2. LASIK complications include: over- or undercorrection, glare/halos at night, dry eye, irregular/poor flap (too thick or thin, button-hole, incomplete, free cap), epithelial defect, decentered ablation, irregular astigmatism, flap dislocation, striae, epithelial ingrowth, interface inflammation (diffuse lamellar keratitis [DLK]), central toxic keratopathy, infection, scarring, and keratectasia. Late DLK may occur (any time in the future) after a corneal abrasion.

3. Stage 2 DLK, which requires frequent topical steroids. Steroid eye drops should be prescribed initially every hour while awake and steroid ointment at bedtime. The eye should be checked daily for improvement, and the steroids are tapered as the DLK resolves. If the interface inflammation progresses to stage 3 or 4, then the flap should be lifted and the stromal bed irrigated. A short course of oral steroids may also be given.

A 50-year-old man reports a history of radial keratotomy (RK) surgery 20 years ago. He has noted glare and starbursts at night since the surgery. He used to experience fluctuating vision but says this has improved. He also notes that his vision has gradually deteriorated, especially over the last 10 years, and he needs stronger glasses for better reading as well as distance vision.

1. What would you specifically look for on examination?
2. What would you tell him about his symptoms and what are the treatment options?

1. Manifest refraction, pupil size in dim and bright light, the corneal status (number of RK incisions and optical zone size, central irregularity, scarring, dryness), presence of cataract and macular pathology. If there is visual fluctuation throughout the day, then morning and afternoon refractions should be performed.

2. Glare/starbursts are common after RK, particularly with smaller optical zones. The deep radial corneal incisions change the shape of the cornea but also weaken the cornea and can produce fluctuations in vision throughout the day and from day to day as refractive shifts occur. Altitude and humidity changes can exacerbate the fluctuations. Over time, many RK patients develop a progressive hyperopic shift (PERK study 10-year results found 43% of patients had at least a 1 D shift). In addition, this patient is presbyopic and is noting the combined effect of progressive hyperopia from the RK plus increasing presbyopia.

   Treatment options include: correction of any refractive error, and pharmacologic (alphagan or pilocarpine) to reduce pupil size and decrease nighttime glare/starburst. He may need different glasses for different times of the day depending on the amount of fluctuation. If the refractive error is stable, then surface ablation can be performed with topical mitomycin C (to prevent scarring). If his symptoms are due to a cataract, then cataract surgery should be discussed and the patient informed that the refractive outcome is less predictable because of his previous RK surgery (eg, accurately measuring central corneal power), and therefore he may require a second procedure (laser vision correction, piggyback IOL, or IOL exchange) to correct a significant residual refractive error.

Power: 42.7D
(7.91 mm)
From vertex:
Dist 0.00 mm
S-merid 0°

SimK Values:

43.75D @80
41.62D @170

OD

08/05/09
9:32 AM

Axial Map

Power: 42.9D
(7.87 mm)
From vertex:
Dist 0.00 mm
S-merid 0°

SimK Values:

44.75D @80
40.25D @170

OS

08/05/09
9:32 AM

Axial Map

A patient with astigmatism complains of problems adapting to her new glasses and says she can see better with her old glasses. Her old prescription is $-5.00 + 2.00 \times 85$ OD and $-6.50 + 3.50 \times 85$ OS; her new prescription is $-5.25 + 2.25 \times 95$ OD and $-7.50 + 4.25 \times 80$ OS.

1. How would you address her complaint?
2. What does the corneal topography show?
3. What is the typical natural history of corneal astigmatism?

1. The new glasses should be measured with a lensometer to confirm that the prescription is correct, the ocular alignment of the lenses checked, and the visual acuity recorded. The manifest refraction should then be rechecked carefully, and consider performing a cycloplegic refraction. If there is an error in the glasses or lens alignment, then simply remaking the lenses may resolve the problem. If the repeat manifest or cycloplegic refraction is different from the glasses prescription, then a new prescription should be given to the patient. Finally, patients with large levels of correction are particularly sensitive to small changes in their glasses prescription (ie, >0.50 D and/or >5° axis rotation), and the vertex distance and base curve of the lenses must also be taken into account. Therefore it may be necessary to make only a small change in the prescription at a time until the full change can be tolerated. When there is a significant change in the prescription the patient should be told of this and warned that it may take some time to adapt to the new glasses.

2. The corneal topography demonstrates regular with-the-rule astigmatism, which appears as a vertically oriented symmetric bowtie. According to the SimK values, there is 2.13 D of astigmatism in the 80 degree meridian OD and 4.50 D of astigmatism in the 80 degree meridian OS.

3. Corneal astigmatism tends to be with-the-rule in children and typically decreases with age. Adults tend to have against-the-rule astigmatism that increases with age. Approximately 50% of the population has 0.75 D or more of astigmatism.

A 38-year-old myopic woman complains that her bulky, heavy glasses are a nuisance and she would like to investigate other options.

1. What are the alternatives and what other information would you like to know?

Additional information: she has worn glasses for 30 years, the last change was 7 years ago, she is not interested in contact lenses, has no other eye problems, and has not noticed a recent change in vision. Her current glasses are −7.25 +1.00×100 OD and −8.00+2.50×20 OS, her vision with these glasses is 20/20 OU, her refraction yields the same prescription and vision. There is no evident anterior or posterior segment abnormality on slit-lamp exam and ophthalmoscopy. She is interested in refractive surgery.

2. What surgical options are available and what tests would you perform?

Additional information: corneal pachymetry is thinnest centrally and measures 505 μm OD and 510 μm OS, angles are open/grade 4 OU, anterior chamber depth is 3.5 mm OD and 3.6 mm OS, and endothelial cell count is normal OU. Her corneal topography shows:

3. How do you interpret the topography maps, and how do the new data affect her surgical options?
4. What are the complications of phakic IOL implantation?

1. Depending on her refractive error her options include: new glasses with high index lenses, contact lenses, and refractive surgery. It would be important to know more about her ocular history and exam. Specifically, when did she start wearing glasses, when was her last prescription change, has she tried contact lenses, and if so what type, for how long, and what did she think about them? Does she have any other past ocular history? Has her vision changed recently? How do the glasses interfere with her lifestyle, daily activities, and hobbies? Has she thought about refractive surgery and, if so, what does she hope to accomplish? With regard to the eye exam, what is her current prescription, visual acuity with correction, and manifest refraction? Are there any abnormalities on exam?

2. Possible surgical options are laser vision correction, phakic IOL, and refractive lens exchange (RLE). However, the disadvantages of RLE are the loss of accommodation and greater risk of vision-threatening complications due to more invasive surgery. To assist in deciding which option is most appropriate, it is necessary to obtain corneal topography, pachymetry, gonioscopy, anterior chamber depth, and endothelial cell evaluation.

3. The CVK reveals form fruste keratoconus OD and mild pellucid marginal degeneration OS, and her corneas are thin, so she is not a candidate for laser vision correction. Her surgical options are lens procedures: phakic IOL or RLE. Since she has a stable refraction and excellent vision with glasses at age 38 years old, it is unlikely that her corneas will change significantly. If she desires phakic IOL surgery, a toric design should be considered to correct her astigmatism OS since corneal astigmatic procedures (corneal-relaxing incisions and laser vision correction) should not be performed. However, a small amount of residual ametropia could possibly be corrected with photorefractive keratectomy (PRK) particularly after corneal collagen cross linking. Similarly, if she prefers RLE, then toric presbyopia-correcting lenses or toric monofocal IOLs set for monovision should be considered, otherwise she will require glasses for the presbyopia or astigmatism.

4. The main risks are corneal endothelial cell loss, glaucoma, iritis, and cataract. The risk of these complications varies depending on the style of IOL:

5. Angle-supported: highest risk of corneal endothelial damage; may also develop glaucoma.

6. Iris-supported: highest risk of iris damage, iritis, and IOL dislocation.

7. Posterior chamber: highest risk of cataract and angle-closure glaucoma.

8. Furthermore, there is a small risk of lens decentration/dislocation, infection, cystoid macular edema, retinal detachment, and disruption of the anterior lens capsule.

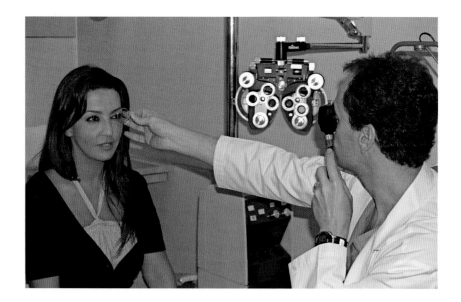

A 34-year-old woman broke her glasses and wants a new prescription. She does not have any old records or glasses to measure.

1. Describe the technique of streak retinoscopy.
2. What methods can be used for an irregular cornea?

1. Retinoscopy is a method of objectively measuring the refractive state of an eye. With a phoropter or free lenses, the examiner moves the light streak across the pupil and changes the correcting lenses until the reflex movement is neutralized (pupil appears uniformly illuminated). This occurs at the far point. If the far point is between the examiner and patient (myopic), the reflex moves in the direction opposite to the retinoscope sweep ("against" motion). If the far point is behind the examiner (hyperopia), the reflex has "with" motion. The final refraction is then determined by adjusting for the working distance (add reciprocal of working distance to the final finding).

2. For a scissoring reflex, which occurs in keratoconus, observe the central area of the reflex. If the reflex is poor or irregular, then alternate methods should be used, such as a contact lens overrefraction or stenopeic slit refraction.

A 73-year-old man reports blurry vision especially in his right eye. He says he was told he has cataracts but wants a second opinion about surgery. His old glasses are −3.00 + 0.75 × 180 OU and he says he used to have equal vision in both eyes. On examination, you find his manifest refraction is −6.25 + 2.00 × 15 OD and −5.00 + 1.00 × 180 OS giving BSCVA (Best Spectacle-Corrected Visual Acuity) of 20/70 OD and 20/25 OS. There is a 4 + nuclear sclerotic/2 + posterior subcapsular cataract OD and a 4 + nuclear sclerotic cataract OS. The rest of the eye exam is normal.

1. What additional information would be helpful?
2. How would you advise this patient regarding cataract surgery?

1. More information about the history and symptoms would be helpful: How long has he been having trouble with his vision? How does the reduced vision interfere with his activities (ie, reading, driving, watching TV, computer work, hobbies, glare/halo/starbursts, etc.)? What are his activities/hobbies and how has he used glasses or contact lenses in the past?

    Results of pinhole vision and PAM (potential acuity meter) for OD, and BAT (brightness acuity [glare] test) for OS would be helpful for determining visual potential OD and visual significance of the cataract OS.

2. This patient has a visually significant cataract OD and possibly one OS, and he also has a large myopic shift with anisometropia. The main issues regarding surgery are the desired refractive outcome and timing of surgery OS.

    Refractive outcome: it is important to inquire about the patient's visual needs and preferred use of glasses for various distances. Since he was a low myope, he may like to read or do close work without glasses and doesn't mind wearing glasses for driving, so he may prefer a monofocal IOL targeted for reading vision. On the other hand, he may have always found glasses a nuisance and would like to reduce his dependence on them as much as possible, so he may prefer multifocal/extended depth of focus (EDF)/accommodating IOLs or monovision. Therefore the various IOL options must be discussed thoroughly.

    Timing of surgery OS: it is also necessary to inform the patient about potential problems with anisometropia/aniseikonia and how this can be addressed (ie, contact lens, laser vision correction) if he does not want cataract surgery OS shortly after OD, particularly if he desires full distance correction with cataract surgery OD.

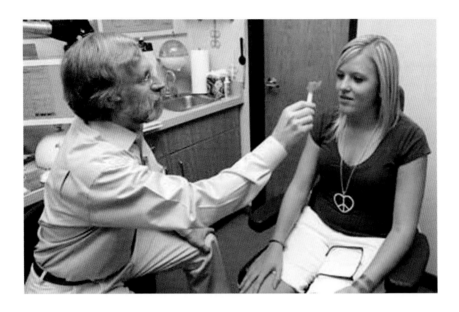

A 23-year-old graduate student complains of headache and eyestrain for the past year. She says her vision has always been fine but a few years ago she was prescribed a pair of reading glasses. They helped only a little, so she wore them occasionally but lost them after a year. Her past ocular history is otherwise unremarkable.

1. What is the differential diagnosis and how would you determine the diagnosis?

Additional information: she has no past medical history and is not taking any medicines. Her manifest refraction is plano OU, cycloplegic refraction is +0.50 D OU, extraocular motility is full, the eyes are orthophoric at distance and there is a 6 PD exophoria at near, accommodative amplitude is normal.

2. What is the diagnosis?
3. How would you treat this patient?

1. The differential diagnosis includes hyperopia, accommodative insufficiency, and convergence insufficiency.

   Accommodative insufficiency is associated with systemic processes such as hypothyroidism, anemia, pregnancy, nutritional deficiencies, and chronic illness, so she should be questioned about her past medical history and current medications. The relevant parts of the eye exam to distinguish among the possible etiologies are: manifest and cycloplegic refractions, ocular alignment and motility, near and far points, accommodative and convergence amplitudes. Hyperopia would be revealed by the refractions (other tests would be normal), and convergence insufficiency would be diagnosed by exophoria greater at near than distance.

2. Convergence insufficiency.

3. Orthoptic exercises to improve fusional amplitudes, such as pencil push-ups, may be helpful. Another option is base-out (BO) prism glasses to stimulate convergence. Rarely is surgery (medial rectus resection) required.

A 51-year-old woman underwent retinal detachment repair with scleral buckle of the right eye 2 weeks ago. Her macula was not affected. She notices that her vision is blurry and she is seeing double. Her uncorrected visual acuity is 20/60 OD and 20/20 OS.

1. What is the most likely cause of her complaints?
2. What single test would help determine the etiology?

Additional information: pinhole improves her vision to 20/20 OD, but does not resolve the diplopia. Her manifest refraction is −2.25+0.75×135 OD and plano OS. She has a right exotropia of 8 PD and hypertropia of 3 PD.

3. How would you manage her?
4. What is the definition of a prism diopter?
5. How are deviations measured with plastic prisms and with glass prisms?
6. How does a minus lens affect the measurement of a tropia?

1. The blurry vision is most likely due to induced myopia (and possible astigmatism) from the scleral buckle, but could be a result of damage from the retinal detachment. The diplopia may also be due to the induced ametropia, but could be caused by strabismus from the scleral buckle.

2. Pinhole vision. If the vision improves, then the blurriness is due to a refractive error. If the diplopia improves then this is also related to the blurry vision and ametropia. If the diplopia does not improve, then an ocular misalignment is present.

3. She should be given her full glasses prescription with prism correction to alleviate the diplopia. Strabismus surgery or buckle removal could be considered in the future.

4. The displacement (in cm) of a light ray passing through a prism, measured 100 cm (1 m) from the prism.

5. Plastic prisms are held with the back surface parallel to the frontal plane. Glass prisms are held in the Prentice position with the back surface perpendicular to the visual axis. The apex of the prism is pointed in the direction of the eye deviation (ie, base-in for exotropia). Stacking prisms is not additive, but holding prisms in front of each eye is.

6. Minus measures more. Minus lenses make the deviation appear larger; plus lenses decrease the measured deviation. The prismatic effect of glasses on strabismic deviations is calculated as follows: $2.5 \times D = \%$ difference.

An angry patient walks into your office complaining that the new distance glasses you prescribed are terrible. He has tried them for 2 weeks and cannot get used to them. The glasses make him feel sick. There was only a minor change (0.25 D) in the prescription compared with his old glasses.

1. What do you do?

Additional information: the glasses were made correctly; he says his vision is clear when he looks straight ahead, but everything seems more magnified and his vision is distorted when he looks to the sides; he cannot do anything to make it better. The PD is right, the optical centers are placed correctly, and repeat refraction is the same as the prescription you recently gave him.

2. What else should you check and how?

1. It is important to explain to the patient that there are a number of reasons why he may be having difficulty with the glasses and you will take care of the problem. First, the glasses should be measured with a lensometer to determine whether they were made correctly. If they were, the patient should be questioned about his symptoms: is the vision clear or blurry, is there any distortion, is the difficulty in one eye or both eyes? Can he make it better by adjusting the glasses or moving or turning his eyes or head? Check the ocular alignment of the lenses and repeat the manifest refraction.

2. The base curve of the lenses should be checked with a Geneva lens clock because a change in base curve can cause these symptoms (distortion and the feeling of motion sickness when looking off-center). Increasing the base curve also results in thicker lenses, and more magnification occurs.

A 16-year-old aphakic girl is interested in wearing contact lenses instead of aphakic glasses. Her manifest refraction is +10.50 + 1.00 × 90 OD and +11.25 + 0.50 × 90 OS.

1. What are the disadvantages of aphakic spectacles?

2. What would the image magnification be with a contact lens, and with an IOL?

3. What are her contact lens options?

4. Would the power of the contact lenses she requires be stronger or weaker than her glasses prescription? Why?

1. The disadvantages of aphakic glasses are: image magnification of 25%, altered depth perception, pincushion distortion, ring scotoma (prismatic effect at edge of lens causes visual field loss of 20%), and the "jack-in-the-box" phenomenon (peripherally invisible objects suddenly appear when gaze is shifted).

2. 7% enlargement with contact lens and 2.5% with IOL.

3. She could wear soft lenses (spherical OU or possibly a toric lens OD for sharper vision) or rigid gas permeable lenses OU (which will provide sharper vision by correcting her astigmatism).

4. Because of the difference in vertex distance between glasses and contact lens, the power of the required correcting lens is different. The effectivity of a plus lens increases as it moves further from the eye (greater plus power), whereas the lens effectivity of a minus lens increases as it moves closer to the eye. The more powerful the lens, the more significant is the change in position. As any lens moves closer to the nodal point of the eye, more plus power is required to keep the image focused onto the retina. Therefore the contact lens this patient needs has more plus power than her glasses lens. The power is determined from:

   1. Focal point of original lens = far point.

   2. Distance of new lens from far point = required focal length of new lens.

   3. Power of new lens = reciprocal of new focal length.

      This can be approximated with the formula: $D_2 = D_1 + S(D_1)^2$ (where S = vertex distance in meters).

A 76-year-old woman with macular degeneration reports more difficulty with her vision over the past few months. She used to be able to read large print books with bright light but is struggling to do so now, so she wants to get new reading glasses. Her visual acuity is 20/400 OD and 20/80 OS. She denies any change in appearance of the Amsler grid, which she checks several times a week OS, and exam of the maculas shows a disciform scar OD and drusen with retinal pigment epithelium (RPE) atrophy OS.

1. How would you estimate the add power for reading glasses?
2. What type of low-vision aids would be helpful for this patient?

1. Kestenbaum's rule can be used to estimate the strength of the plus lens required to read newspaper print without accommodation. This is useful in patients with low vision. The necessary add power is the reciprocal of the best distance acuity. This patient has no central vision OD and uses her left eye for reading. Therefore she would need a reading add of +4.00 D (ie, 80/20) for a working distance of 0.25 m (the reciprocal of the add power). This should be checked and refined with trial frames or a phoropter.

2. If the new reading glasses are not sufficient, then other options include spectacle-mounted magnifiers (telescopes for distance or microscopes for near), handheld or stand magnifiers and telescopes, video magnifiers (CCTVs), electronic reading machines, and talking appliances. The patient may benefit from a low-vision consultation to assess her visual needs and try various aids to determine what works best for her.

A 53-year-old woman is unhappy with her current contacts and wants to be fitted for new lenses.

1. What is the technique for fitting a rigid gas permeable (RGP) contact lens?
2. What is the technique for fitting a soft contact lens (SCL)?
3. The RGP lens rides high; how can the lens parameters be changed to improve the fit?

1. RGPs are fitted using the SAM-FAP rule ("steeper add minus, flatter add plus"). The contact lens is fitted steeper than the average corneal keratometry measurement. This forms a plus tear meniscus between the cornea and RGP lens, which alters the required power of the lens. Therefore it is necessary to subtract power (add minus) at the end of the power calculation. For each diopter the base curve is made "steeper than K", subtract 1 D from the final lens power. If the lens is fit flatter than K, then a minus tear meniscus is formed, so it is necessary to add plus power at the end of the calculation. A contact lens overrefraction is performed to determine the necessary power. If a trial lens is not available for overrefraction, then the power calculation is performed as follows:

   1. Measure refraction and keratometry.
   2. Choose base curve steeper than flat K (usually +0.50 D steeper to form a tear lens; tear lens prevents apical touch).
   3. Convert refraction to minus cylinder form and zero vertex distance; disregard the cylinder (minus cylinder is formed by the tears).
   4. Power of contact lens is sphere from refraction adjusted for tear lens (subtract +0.50); "SAM-FAP".

   To evaluate the fit, assess the fluorescein pattern, lens movement, and centration.

2. The power of a SCL is based on the spherical equivalent manifest refraction corrected for vertex distance. The base curve is based on average keratometry measurements. To evaluate the fit, assess the movement of the lens. Poor movement means the lens is too tight (too steep) and excessive movement indicates that the lens is too flat.

3. The lens is too tight, so to loosen it either increase the radius of curvature or decrease the diameter.

Condensing lenses are used with an indirect ophthalmoscope to examine the retina.

1. What are the advantages of the indirect ophthalmoscope?
2. What are the different types of magnification?
3. What is the retinal magnification with a 20 D lens?

1. Larger field of view and stereopsis compared with the direct ophthalmoscope. Field of view is 25° (versus 7°) and magnification is 2–3× (versus 15×).

2. Transverse, axial, and angular magnification.

   Transverse (linear or lateral): magnification of image size (away from the optical axis). Equal to the ratio of image height to object height ($M_L = I/O$).

   Axial: magnification of depth (along the optical axis). Equal to the square of the transverse magnification ($M_{Ax} = M_L^2$).

   Angular: magnification of angle subtended by an image with respect to an object. Used when the object or image size cannot be measured. ($M_A = D/4$, standardized to 25 cm [¼ m], the near point of the average eye.)

3. $M_A = D_{eye}/D_{lens} = 60/20 = 3\times$.

A 34-year-old man with a corneal scar and best spectacle corrected visual acuity of 20/100 in his right eye wants to know if his vision can be improved.

1. How would you evaluate him?
2. If this patient has better visual potential, what are the surgical options?

1. A number of tests can be performed to determine the visual potential including pinhole acuity, RGP contact lens overrefraction, and potential acuity meter (PAM) test. Visual evoked response (VER) could also be performed.

2. Depending on the location, size, and depth of the scar, the options are phototherapeutic keratectomy (PTK), rotational corneal autograft, penetrating keratoplasty, anterior lamellar keratoplasty (ALK), and deep lamellar keratoplasty (DLK).

A 68-year-old man who underwent cataract surgery 1 month ago complains of blurred vision since surgery. On exam, his uncorrected vision is 20/100 at distance and J1 at near in the operated eye. He is unhappy because he expected good distance vision without glasses and would like to wear glasses to read.

1. What is the problem?
2. What are the possible etiologies?
3. What are the surgical treatment options?

1. Myopic refractive outcome.

2. A refractive surprise after cataract surgery occurs because the IOL is the wrong power or is in the wrong position. Wrong IOL power is due to an error in axial length measurement, error in keratometry measurement, use of an incorrect IOL calculation formula, or insertion of the wrong IOL. Wrong IOL position is due to sulcus placement without reducing the IOL power, and anterior displacement of an IOL in the bag from a large capsulorhexis, capsular distension/capsular block syndrome, capsular contraction, or upside-down placement of an angulated IOL.

3. This patient can be treated with IOL exchange, piggyback IOL, and laser vision correction. For capsular block syndrome, a Nd:YAG laser anterior capsulotomy should be performed to release the trapped fluid and allow the IOL to return to its normal position.

1. What is the name of the test depicted in the photo?

2. How does this test work and how is it performed?

1. The duochrome test.

2. The duochrome test uses the principle of chromatic aberration to monocularly refine the spherical endpoint and check the accuracy and balance of the refraction. Light of shorter wavelengths is refracted more than light of longer wavelengths (green is bent more than red and is therefore focused anterior to red). The green and red filters create a 0.5 D difference. The patient must therefore have 20/30 or better visual acuity in order to distinguish the difference. If the patient sees the letters on the green side of the chart clearer then the focal point is behind the retina (the eye is overminused) and plus sphere is added to the prescription. If the patient sees the red side clearer then the focal point is in front of the retina (the eye is overplussed) and minus sphere is added to the prescription. This can be remembered with the mnemonic RAM-GAP (**R**ed **A**dd **M**inus - **G**reen **A**dd **P**lus). The technique is to start with the red side clearer and add minus sphere in 0.25 D steps until the letters on the red and green sides are of equal clarity (ie, the red and green light are the same distance (0.25 D) behind and in front of the retina, respectively), then the focal point is on the retina and the prescription is balanced. The duochrome test works in colorblind patients because it uses chromatic aberration not color discrimination.

1. What device is shown and how does it work?

2. What are the limitations of this device?

3. What is the astigmatic effect from the posterior corneal surface?

1. A keratometer. This device measures the curvature of the anterior corneal surface based on the power of a reflecting surface. It does this by measuring the size of an image reflected from 2 paracentral points and utilizes doubling prisms to stabilize the image enabling more accurate focusing. The anterior corneal curvature is then calculated using the convex mirror formula, and the corneal power is estimated empirically based on Snell's law of refraction with simplified optics. The keratometer adjusts the index of refraction (1.3375 vs. 1.376) to account for the posterior corneal power and also to allow 45 D to equal 7.5 mm radius of curvature (K (diopters) = 337.5/r).

2. Limitations of the keratometer include: it only measures a small region of the cornea (2 points at the 3–4 mm zone), it does not provide information about the cornea central or peripheral to these points, it measures different regions for corneas of different powers, it assumes the cornea is spherocylindrical and symmetric with a major and minor axis separated by 90 degrees, it ignores spherical aberration, it is susceptible to focusing and misalignment errors, and it cannot accurately measure irregular corneas.

3. The posterior corneal surface contributes approximately 0.4 D of against-the-rule astigmatism to the total corneal power. This is important when determining the amount of corneal astigmatic correction during cataract surgery and refractive lens exchange.

1. Name the various types of gonioscopy lenses and explain how they differ.

2. Define the critical angle.

3. What is total internal reflection and how is this relevant to the eye exam?

1. There are a variety of gonioscopy lenses: Koeppe-style lenses (ie, Koeppe, Barkan, Wurst, Swan-Jacob, and Richardson) for direct gonioscopy (direct and upright view of the iridocorneal angle structures with a binocular microscope, light source, and supine patient, usually in the operating room), and the Goldmann-style lenses and the 4- or 6-mirror lenses (ie, Zeiss, Posner, Sussman) for indirect gonioscopy (indirect and inverted view of the opposite angle with the slit lamp biomicroscope and patient sitting upright).

    The Goldmann lenses typically contain three mirrors, but there are lenses with only one mirror. The lens rests on the sclera, vaults over the cornea and therefore requires a viscous coupling solution (ie, Goniosol), and cannot be used for indentation gonioscopy. In the three-mirrors lenses, each mirror has a different angulation to view different parts of the eye: the angle (~60 degrees), peripheral retina (~65 degrees), and mid-peripheral retina (~75 degrees). The center of the lens can be used to visualize the posterior pole. Because only one of the mirrors can be used for angle viewing, the lens must be rotated 360 degrees to examine the entire angle.

    The 4- and 6-mirror lenses are composed of symmetric mirrors with the same angulation (~60–63 degrees) so that the angle structures can be viewed with minimal or no rotation of the lens. These lenses rest on the cornea without the need for a coupling solution. This enables the examiner to perform indentation gonioscopy to differentiate between appositional and synechial angle closure. Appositional angle closure opens with indentation of the central cornea, which pushes aqueous peripherally, and synechial angle closure does not open with indentation.

2. The critical angle is the angle at which incident light is bent 90 degrees away from the normal (when going from a medium of higher to lower index of refraction (n)) and after which all light is reflected. The critical angle differs for different interfaces and depends upon the indices of refraction of the material on either side of the interface. The critical angle of the cornea (air/cornea interface) is 46.5 degrees.

3. Total internal reflection is an optical phenomenon that occurs when the angle of incidence exceeds the critical angle. This causes light to be reflected back into the material with higher index of refraction. Angle structures cannot be directly visualized owing to total internal reflection at the air/cornea interface. Therefore a gonioscopy lens is required to view the angle structures.

A 72-year-old woman has a +2.00 D refractive surprise after cataract surgery and desires a piggyback intraocular lens (IOL) procedure.

1. How is the correct piggyback IOL power calculated, and what power does this patient require for emmetropia?
2. What are the necessary considerations when planning to perform a piggyback IOL procedure?

1. As a general guideline, to correct myopia the necessary IOL power is 1.2 times the myopic refractive error, and to correct hyperopia the necessary IOL power is 1.5 times the hyperopic refractive error. The Holladay R formula can also be used to calculate the appropriate power for a piggyback IOL. In this case a +3.00 D IOL should be used to achieve emmetropia.

2. The relevant considerations for piggyback IOL procedures are the IOL power, material, edge design, and position. IOLs with low negative or low positive dioptric power are required. The material should be different from that of the existing IOL in the eye (ie, acrylic vs. silicone) to minimize the risk of an intralenticular membrane formation. The piggyback lens is placed in the ciliary sulcus and should have a rounded (not square) edge, a posterior angulation, and a 3-piece design with sufficient overall length in order to prevent pigment dispersion and iris damage from chafing the posterior iris surface.

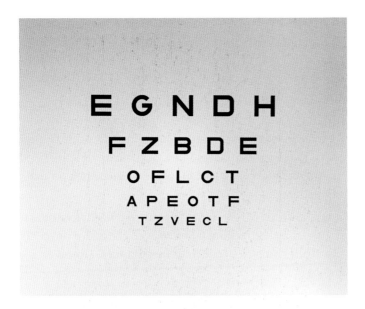

1. What is Snellen acuity and what does Snellen notation mean?
2. What are the characteristics of the ETDRS chart?

3. What is the principle of a pinhole?
4. What is the optimal size of a pinhole and why?

1. Snellen acuity refers to the standard 20/20 notation of measuring visual acuity and is based on the angle that the smallest letter subtends on the retina. The numerator refers to the testing distance (ie, 20 feet or 6 meters); the denominator represents the distance at which a letter subtends 5 minutes of arc (ie, 20/40 letter subtends 5 minutes at 40 feet, 20/20 letter subtends 5 minutes at 20 feet), or the distance at which a person with normal vision can see the letters. Each stroke width and space subtends 1 minute of arc.

2. The Early Treatment Diabetic Retinopathy Study (ETDRS) visual acuity measurement was designed to eliminate the inaccuracies of other tests and is considered the gold standard for population studies and clinical research. The ETDRS chart is characterized by a proportional layout and geometric progression of letter sizes. The chart consists of five letters per line, the space between letters is equal to the size of the letters on that line, and the optotype height changes in 0.1 log unit increments.

3. A pinhole allows only the undeviated paraxial light rays to focus on the retina. It reduces refractive error and improves vision by increasing depth of focus, but it is limited by diffraction. A pinhole can correct for up to 3 D of refractive error and can also improve vision in eyes with corneal or lenticular irregularities. However, a pinhole can reduce vision in eyes with retinal disorders.

4. The optimal size of a pinhole is 1.2 mm. A smaller hole limits visual acuity because of increased diffraction and reduced amount of light entering the eye.

A 60-year-old woman says she needs a pressure check. She has been treated for glaucoma for 3 years with a prostaglandin analog in both eyes. Her vision is 20/25 OU, intraocular pressure (IOP) is 14 mmHg OU, and she has a stable superior arcuate visual field (VF) defect in the left eye. Her right optic nerve head appears normal and her left optic nerve (ON) head is depicted below:

1. What does her optic nerve photo show?

2. What is the pathophysiology?

3. What tests can be used to confirm the diagnosis?

4. How would you manage this patient?

5. What are the potential complications of optic nerve drusen?

1. Optic nerve head drusen (pseudopapilledema).

2. Superficial or buried hyaline bodies in the prelaminar optic nerve that have become calcified.

3. B-scan ultrasound, CT scan, or autofluorescence.

4. It is important to determine whether this patient's VF defect is due to glaucoma or the ON head drusen. Therefore it would be helpful to obtain her old records to know what old field tests showed, what her maximum eye pressure was, and whether her optic nerve appearance has changed. If she never had elevated IOP or progression of the scotoma or optic cupping, then the glaucoma diagnosis may be suspect and it is reasonable to stop the glaucoma drop and follow her IOP. A diurnal curve may also be useful for determining her maximum IOP. If previous records are unavailable, then new baselines should be established with visual fields, gonioscopy, corneal pachymetry, and optic nerve head images.

5. Optic nerve drusen can cause VF defects (typically enlarged blind spot, arcuate scotoma, or sectoral scotoma that is stable/nonprogressive), anterior ischemic optic neuropathy, choroidal neovascularization, subretinal or vitreous hemorrhage, and vascular occlusion.

A 70-year-old man reports intermittent double vision for the past week and is panicked because of blurry vision in the right eye for 2 days. He says his vision has been excellent since his cataract surgery several years earlier. He takes medication for hypertension and high cholesterol. Ocular exam shows visual acuity of 20/200 OD and 20/25 OS. There is a positive relative afferent pupillary defect (RAPD) in the right eye, extraocular motility is full, and anterior segment exam reveals well-positioned posterior chamber IOLs. The retina is within normal limits and the right optic nerve is pictured above.

1. What are you concerned about and what further history would you obtain?
2. How would you work up this patient?
3. What treatment would you prescribe if this patient has giant cell arteritis (GCA), and what is the prognosis?
4. What is Foster–Kennedy syndrome and pseudo-Foster–Kennedy syndrome?

1. The history and findings are suggestive of anterior ischemic optic neuropathy (AION). It is important to distinguish between the arteritic (GCA) and nonarteritic (NAION) forms because the arteritic form must be treated to prevent visual loss in the fellow eye. NAION is most often spontaneous but is associated with hypertension, diabetes, ischemic heart disease, hypercholesterolemia, and smoking. This patient has increased blood pressure and cholesterol, but it cannot be assumed that his optic neuropathy is nonarteritic. The patient must be asked about the characteristic symptoms of GCA: headache, scalp tenderness, jaw claudication (pain with chewing), weight loss, fever, and anorexia, as well as neck pain, eye pain, diplopia, joint pain (symptoms of polymyalgia rheumatica), and history of anemia.

2. A stat erythrocyte sedimentation rate (ESR; sed rate) is required to rule out arteritic AION. An elevated ESR is considered to be $> (age/2)$ for males and $> ([age + 10]/2)$ for females. Other labs that should be ordered are C-reactive protein (elevated CRP [>2.45 mg/dL]) and complete blood count (CBC) (low hematocrit, high platelets). Fluorescein angiography shows choroidal nonperfusion in the arteritic form. Some physicians routinely obtain a temporal artery biopsy (sometimes bilateral) on all patients, which should be performed within 2 weeks of initiating steroid treatment. Because of skip lesions, the biopsy specimen should be at least 3 cm in length.

3. Emergent treatment with high-dose steroids (prednisone 60–120 mg orally; consider IV initially [1 g qd for 3 days]), which should not be delayed while waiting for the temporal artery biopsy. Unfortunately, treatment does not improve the outcome in the affected eye but is necessary to prevent visual loss in the fellow eye (65% risk of involvement without treatment; however, some patients lose vision despite treatment). Patients should be followed by an internist and/or rheumatologist to monitor the response to therapy and to slowly taper the steroids. GCA is also associated with other ocular and systemic complications: retinal artery occlusion, ophthalmic artery occlusion, anterior segment ischemia, cranial nerve palsy (especially CN 6), and stroke.

4. Foster–Kennedy syndrome is a frontal lobe mass (usually meningioma) that causes anosmia, ipsilateral optic atrophy from tumor compression, and contralateral optic nerve edema from elevated intracranial pressure. The same optic nerve findings (disc edema in one eye and disc pallor in the other eye) can occur in bilateral AION, which is called pseudo-Foster–Kennedy syndrome.

A 45-year-old woman reports double vision that started this morning after breakfast. She also notices that her eyelid seems droopy. She has mild hypertension and says her blood pressure has been stable for years on medication.

1. What findings are seen in the photo?
2. What other history would you ask the patient?

Additional information: the patient says that she has a headache but she often gets headaches, although this seems worse and has not improved significantly with ibuprofen. She denies any trauma. On exam her vision is 20/20 OU, there is a right upper eyelid ptosis, and the right eye is turned down and out. The right pupil is large and poorly reactive to light. Other cranial nerves are intact. Intraocular pressure is 18 mmHg, and the rest of the anterior and posterior segment exams are normal.

3. What are the diagnosis and possible etiologies?
4. What would your next step be?
5. How would your treatment differ if this patient were older than age 50 with an isolated pupil-sparing third nerve palsy?

1. This patient has a right upper eyelid ptosis, ocular misalignment, and anisocoria with a larger right pupil.

2. The patient should be asked about headache and a history of trauma or cancer.

3. This patient has a pupil-involving CN 3 palsy OD. Despite a history of hypertension, she is young and has pupil involvement, and pain. It is therefore most important to rule out a posterior communicating artery aneurysm, which is a neurosurgical emergency. It is unlikely to be due to other etiologies such as microvascular (diabetes, hypertension), trauma (no history of this), tumor, or infection.

4. Urgent neuroimaging with magnetic resonance imaging (MRI), magnetic resonance angiography (MRA)/computed tomography angiography (CTA), or both.

5. Older patients with isolated pupil-sparing 3rd nerve palsies should be observed carefully for pupil involvement during the first week, but generally such cases are due to microvascular disease (80% are pupil sparing) and resolve spontaneously in 3 months. Workup is performed if the pupil becomes involved, there is a history of cancer, there are other neurologic abnormalities, or the palsy does not resolve after 3 months. The diplopia can be treated by occluding the paretic eye.

A 55-year-old man reports double vision for a week. He wears bifocals and has had no other change in vision. Exam shows 20/30 vision, normal pupillary responses, mild cataracts, and normal posterior segments in both eyes. Results of ocular motility testing are depicted in the photo.

1. What abnormality does this patient have?

2. What are the possible etiologies?

3. What additional history is pertinent?

Additional information: this is the first time he has had double vision. His past ocular history is negative. He does have diabetes, which is controlled with oral medication.

4. What workup and treatment are required?

1. The patient has an esotropia in primary gaze and deficiency of abduction OS. This is consistent with a lateral rectus (CN 6) palsy.

2. Most commonly it is vasculopathic in adults, but other etiologies include trauma, temporal arteritis, infection, multiple sclerosis, cerebrovascular accidents, increased intracranial pressure, and, rarely, tumors. Other conditions in the differential diagnosis of CN 6 palsy are thyroid-related ophthalmopathy, orbital pseudotumor (idiopathic orbital inflammatory disease), myasthenia gravis, convergence spasm, strabismus, medial orbital wall fracture, and orbital myositis.

3. Has he ever had previous episodes of diplopia or neurologic symptoms? Any previous eye problems, surgery, or trauma? Is the double vision constant, intermittent, or variable? Any medical conditions, specifically hypertension, diabetes, cancer? Any weakness, fatigue, difficulty breathing/swallowing, hoarseness?

4. Treatment of CN 6 palsy depends on the underlying etiology. This is presumably an ischemic isolated mononeuropathy due to diabetes, which is self-limited and should resolve within 3 months so a workup is not necessary. The patient should be reassured and told that he can temporarily cover his left glasses lens or patch the left eye to prevent diplopia or use prism glasses. He should be monitored for other neurologic symptoms. If any develop or his condition does not resolve in 3 months, then neuroimaging is indicated. Additional workup to consider is checking BP, lab tests (CBC, ESR [erythrocyte sedimentation rate], VDRL [Venereal Disease Research Laboratory] or RPR [rapid plasma reagin], FTA-ABS [fluorescent treponemal antibody absorption] or MHA-TP [microhemagglutination assay for *Treponema pallidum*], ANA [antinuclear antibody]), lumbar puncture, and Tensilon test.

A 64-year-old man presents to the emergency room (ER) with left-sided facial pain, swollen eyelid, and double vision. He is a low myope with no significant past ocular history. His visual acuity is 20/40 OD and 20/60 OS without correction and extraocular motility in the left eye is restricted in all positions of gaze.

1. What is the differential diagnosis?

2. What other exam findings might be present?

3. How would you work up this patient?

Additional information: the patient's visual acuity with correction is 20/20 OU, there is no RAPD or efferent defect, but he does have anisocoria with a miotic left pupil. He also has a left ptosis, ocular motility is limited in all positions of gaze, and there is decreased facial sensation of the left forehead and cheek.

4. What nerves are involved and where is the pathology?

1. This patient appears to have multiple CN palsies. These can be caused by tumor, infection, inflammation, meningitis, and vascular lesions in the brain stem, subarachnoid space, cavernous sinus, or orbital apex. Other disorders that mimic multiple CN palsies include chronic progressive external ophthalmoplegia (CPEO), myasthenia gravis, multiple sclerosis, Guillain–Barré syndrome, and progressive supranuclear palsy.

2. Depending on the location of the pathology, other cranial nerves and sympathetic nerves may be affected, so a CN exam must be performed with particular attention to best-corrected visual acuity, anisocoria, pupillary response, extraocular motility, lid position, facial sensation, and facial muscle strength. Possible findings include decreased visual acuity and color vision (orbital apex syndrome), ptosis, strabismus, negative forced ductions, decreased facial sensation in CN V_1–V_2 distribution, relative afferent pupillary defect, miosis (Horner's syndrome), and trigeminal (facial) pain. There may also be proptosis, conjunctival injection, chemosis, increased intraocular pressure, bruit, and retinopathy in cases of high-flow arteriovenous fistulas. Fever, lid edema, and signs of facial infection occur in cases of cavernous sinus thrombosis.

3. Head, orbital, and sinus imaging (CT/MRI–MRA) is required to localize the pathology and direct treatment. Lab tests to order include fasting blood glucose, CBC with differential, ESR, VDRL or RPR, FTA–ABS or MHA–TP, ANA, and blood cultures if infection is suspected. Other possible tests include lumbar puncture and Tensilon test.

4. The history and findings reveal involvement of CN 3, 4, V_1, V_2, 6, and sympathetics (Horner's syndrome), which indicate a cavernous sinus lesion. In contrast, orbital apex syndrome involves CN 2 and does not involve V_2 or the sympathetics (ie, CN 2, 3, 4, V_1, and 6).

You are called to see a 52-year-old woman in the ER with a 1-week history of progressive periorbital pain, headache, redness, and swelling.

1. What would you ask this patient?

2. What is the differential diagnosis?

3. What would you look for on exam to distinguish between these two diagnoses?

Additional information: the patient is diabetic and was admitted to the ER with a blood glucose reading of 625 mg/dL. She has decreased acuity, proptosis, and limited extraocular motility.

4. What organisms cause this infection and what are you most concerned about?

Additional information: a biopsy shows:

5. What is the appropriate treatment?

6. What are the possible complications?

1. Is there any history of trauma, surgery, bites/scratches, infection (sinus, dental, systemic), diabetes? Any fever? Does she notice a change in vision or diplopia? Does she have pain with eye movement?

2. Preseptal or orbital cellulitis.

3. Preseptal cellulitis is an infection anterior to the orbital septum and does not affect the globe, whereas orbital cellulitis is an infection extending posterior to the septum and involves the globe (therefore has eye findings – specifically, decreased vision, positive RAPD, restricted ocular motility, proptosis, pain on eye movement, periorbital swelling, chemosis, and optic disc swelling).

4. Orbital cellulitis is most commonly due to Gram-positive bacteria (*Streptococcus* and *Staphylococcus* species) but can also be caused by fungi (Phycomycetes). Mucormycosis, an aggressive infection by Mucor fungi that causes necrosis, vascular thrombosis, and orbital invasion, must be suspected in this case of an immunocompromised patient.

5. This is *Mucor* infection (the histology shows broad nonseptate fungal hyphae and angiothrombosis), a life-threatening condition requiring emergent IV antifungals and surgical debridement. A CT scan should be obtained to evaluate the extent of involvement. The diabetes must be treated and controlled.

6. *Mucor* can cause retinal vascular occlusions and orbital apex syndrome. It may extend intracranially to cause cavernous sinus thrombosis, meningitis, brain abscess, and death.

A 28-year-old woman reports her eyes have been red for the past year and seem bigger.

1. What is the most likely diagnosis?

2. What other ocular findings are associated with this condition?

3. What is the treatment?

4. What are other causes of proptosis in an adult?

5. What tests are helpful in determining the correct diagnosis?

1. Thyroid-related ophthalmopathy (TRO), most commonly Graves'.

2. In addition to proptosis, other findings include: lid signs (lid retraction, lid lag on downgaze, lagophthalmos), restricted extraocular motility (strabismus), exposure (conjunctival hyperemia, keratopathy), and optic nerve compression (optic neuropathy). (The Werner Classification of eye findings in TRO can be remembered with the mnemonic: NO SPECS [**N**o signs or symptoms, **O**nly signs, **S**oft tissue involvement, **P**roptosis, **E**xtraocular muscle involvement, **C**orneal involvement, **S**ight loss (optic nerve compression)].)

3. Dry eye is treated with lubrication, patching/taping/goggles at bedtime, punctal occlusion, and sometimes with tarsorrhaphy. Extreme proptosis causing severe keratopathy or optic nerve compression is treated with orbital decompression. Diplopia can be treated with prism glasses and eventually surgery (rectus recessions when the strabismus is stable for at least 6 months). Steroids and sometimes radiation are used to reduce muscle enlargement. Surgery is performed in a stepwise fashion with orbital decompression first, then strabismus surgery, and finally lid surgery (eyelid recession). The underlying thyroid disease must also be treated.

4. The differential diagnosis of proptosis in an adult includes: orbital pseudotumor (idiopathic orbital inflammatory disease), orbital and lacrimal gland tumors, orbital vasculitis, trauma, cellulitis, arteriovenous fistula, and cavernous sinus thrombosis.

5. A complete eye exam must be performed with attention to visual acuity, color vision, pupils, motility, forced ductions, eyelid position and movement, exophthalmometry, cornea, tonometry (increased IOP in upgaze), and ophthalmoscopy. Check visual fields as a baseline study in early cases and to rule out optic neuropathy in advanced cases. Thyroid function tests (thyroid stimulating hormone [TSH], thyroxine [total and free T_4], and triiodothyronine [T_3]) and thyroid-stimulating immunoglobulin (TSI) should be ordered. Orbital CT scan may show extraocular muscle enlargement with sparing of the tendons (the inferior rectus is most commonly involved, followed by medial, superior, and lateral), in contrast to IOI, in which the tendons are also enlarged.

A 24-year-old man reports blurry vision in the right eye and then the left eye gradually for several weeks. He is hyperopic with no past ocular or medical history. His best-corrected visual acuity is 20/400 OD and 20/200 OS; pupillary response, extraocular motility, and intraocular pressure are normal. Anterior and posterior segment exams are essentially normal. The optic nerve appearance is shown in the figure.

1. What other history would be useful?

Additional information: the patient's grandfather has macular degeneration, both grandparents have cataracts, and an uncle had poor vision for most of his life. He takes vitamins but no medications. He is a social drinker and occasionally smokes a cigar. He has no known toxic exposures and his past medical history is negative.

2. What is the differential diagnosis?
3. What additional tests would you perform?

Additional information: retinal exam is normal, he has centrocecal scotomas, and significant color vision impairment in both eyes.

4. What is the most likely diagnosis?
5. What are the characteristic findings of this disease?
6. What do you tell him about the disease?

1. Is there any family history of eye problems or visual loss (particularly at a young age)? Any medications, alcohol or tobacco use, toxic exposures, or nutritional deficiencies? Does he have a history of infectious diseases or cancer? Any significant radiation exposure?

2. Hereditary or acquired optic neuropathies (compressive, toxic, nutritional, infectious, traumatic, infiltrative, ischemic).

3. Visual fields and color vision.

4. Leber's hereditary optic neuropathy (LHON).

5. The typical appearance is disc hyperemia, peripapillary telangiectatic vessels, tortuous vessels, peripapillary nerve fiber layer edema, and eventually optic disc pallor.

6. LHON is a hereditary optic neuropathy with maternal inheritance, so it is transmitted to all sons (only 50% are affected). Visual loss occurs in the 2nd–3rd decade of life with bilateral sequential loss of vision to worse than 20/200. Unfortunately there is no treatment.

A 56-year-old woman reports progressive decreased vision in her left eye for the past 3 months. Her past ocular history is negative. On exam, her visual acuity is 20/20 OD and 20/100 OS. Extraocular motility is intact, confrontation visual fields (VF) appear full, and there is a positive RAPD in the left eye.

1. What do you notice about the optic nerve?
2. What additional testing would you perform in the office?

Additional information: color vision is normal OD and reduced OS. Her VF shows:

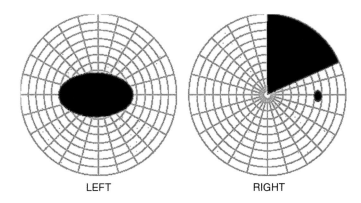

LEFT   RIGHT

3. Does the VF test localize the pathology and, if so, where is the lesion?
4. What is the differential diagnosis?
5. What additional work up is necessary?

1. Optic disc pallor horizontally.

2. VF (tangent screen, Humphrey, or Goldmann) and color vision testing.

3. The VF defect is a junctional scotoma due to a lesion of the optic nerve near the chiasm, which involves the knee of von Willebrand (inferonasal retinal fibers that cross in the chiasm and then travel anteriorly approximately 4 mm into the opposite [contralateral] optic nerve before running posteriorly to the brain) causing central visual loss in the ipsilateral eye and a superotemporal field defect in the contralateral eye.

4. Chiasmal syndrome, which is most commonly a mass lesion but possibly due to hemorrhage. The differential diagnosis includes tumors, pituitary apoplexy, aneurysm, trauma, sarcoidosis, and chiasmal neuritis.

5. Neuroimaging; also consider endocrine evaluation (check hormone levels).

A 22-year-old woman reports decreased vision and eye pain in the left eye that started 2 days ago and has gotten worse. She says everything looks blurry and appears dimmer with that eye.

1. What would you ask this patient?
2. What would you specifically look for on exam?
3. What is the differential diagnosis?

Additional information: she denies any trauma or previous episodes. Her past medical history is negative and she takes only birth control pills. The eye hurts especially when she looks to the right and left. There is no redness, photophobia, or diplopia. She has no other associated symptoms. Her exam is normal except for 20/200 vision and a positive RAPD OS.

4. What is the diagnosis?
5. What additional testing would you perform and why?
6. What are the recommendations for treatment?
7. What is the prognosis?

1. What type of eye pain (foreign body sensation [FBS], sharp, dull, ache, tender to touch, pain with eye movement, headache, periorbital pain)? Any double vision? Any trauma? Any previous episodes? Has the eye been red? Any sensitivity to light? Any other neurologic symptoms? Does she have any medical conditions? Is she taking any medication?

2. On exam, it is important to check the visual acuity, pupillary response with attention to the presence of a RAPD, extraocular motility, cornea, anterior chamber reaction, vitreous, retina, and optic nerve.

3. Corneal lesion (foreign body, abrasion, erosion, ulcer), uveitis, optic neuritis.

4. Retrobulbar optic neuritis.

5. Check color vision, visual fields, and perform a head/orbital MRI to look for periventricular white matter demyelinating lesions or plaques (the best predictor of future development of multiple sclerosis). A neurologic exam should also be performed.

6. According to the Optic Neuritis Treatment Trial (ONTT), if the MRI is positive, then consider systemic steroids (methylprednisolone 250 mg IV q6h for 3 days, followed by prednisone 1 mg/kg/day for 11 days and rapid taper 20 mg/day on day 12 and 10 mg/day on days 13–15). Visual recovery occurred 2 weeks faster with this regimen than with other treatments; however, there was no difference in the final visual acuity. Furthermore, there was a decreased incidence of MS over the next 2 years but there was no difference after 3 years. Oral steroids should not be used alone, because this led to an increased risk of recurrent optic neuritis. Additional treatment recommendations come from the CHAMPS study group, which showed that patients who received weekly intramuscular interferon β-1a (Avonex) after steroid therapy for the first episode of optic neuritis associated with at least two lesions on MRI greater than 3 mm had a reduction in onset of clinical MS over 3 years and improvement or less worsening of MRI lesions.

7. Most patients recover vision over the following months, but the final acuity depends upon the severity of the visual loss. The majority of patients recover 20/20 vision; however, permanent subtle color vision and contrast sensitivity deficits are common. Uhthoff's symptom (blurred vision with increased body temperature or exercise) may occur. Approximately 30% of patients with isolated optic neuritis will experience another attack in either eye, and up to 50% of patients will develop MS over 5–10 years.

A 57-year-old man complains of recent loss of vision. He is a poor historian and tends to ramble. His vague and inconsistent story makes it difficult to elicit an accurate account of his symptoms, but it appears that the decreased vision was sudden and painless. His eye exam is normal except for visual acuity of 20/400 OU.

1. What do you suspect may be the problem and what other questions might be helpful?

2. What tests could you perform to confirm your suspicion?

Additional information: you determine that this patient has hysteria.

3. What strategies can you use to help him "recover" his vision?

1. This case is suspicious for functional visual loss (ie, malingering, hysteria). Malingering is the fabrication of a disorder for secondary gain (usually financial), whereas hysteria is a subconscious expression of symptoms. In order to distinguish between them and rule out any organic disease, it would be helpful to ask about any injuries, medical problems, medications, and social history with particular attention to employment status, stresses, and alcohol/drug use.

2. Carefully performing a variety of vision tests to trick the patient can usually uncover functional visual loss because of inconsistent results. These include distance and near, monocular and binocular, varying the test distance, fogging, red–green glasses with duochrome test or Worth 4 dot test, prism dissociation, stereopsis, startle reflex, proprioception, name signing, mirror tracking, and optokinetic nystagmus response. Visual fields may show unusual patterns such as tunnel vision, spiraling fields, and crossing isopters. Finally, in difficult cases electrophysiologic testing, optical coherence tomography (OCT), fluorescein angiography, or neuroimaging may be necessary.

3. It is helpful to acknowledge the decreased vision and then offer reassurance and a potential way out such as administering a topical medication in the office and then retesting, or having the patient return in several weeks for a repeat examination. Psychiatry consultation is usually not required.

A 58-year-old man presents with a droopy eyelid. He denies any change in vision.

1. What do you notice in the picture?
2. What is the most likely diagnosis?
3. What are the etiologies?
4. What additional history and findings would be helpful?

Additional information: the patient denies any trauma and has no other symptoms. He does not have blurry vision or diplopia. On exam, his vision is 20/20 in both eyes, there is a right upper eyelid ptosis. The eyes are aligned and ocular motility is full. The right pupil is smaller than the left and there is no relative afferent or efferent pupillary defect. Cranial nerves are intact. The rest of the anterior and posterior segment exams are normal.

5. What is the differential diagnosis of anisocoria?
6. What type of pupil testing would you perform?

1. The patient has a right upper eyelid ptosis and anisocoria with a smaller right pupil.

2. Horner's syndrome.

3. The etiology depends upon which neuron is affected: central causes include cerebrovascular accident, neck trauma, tumor, cervical disc disease, and demyelinating disease. These rarely result in an isolated Horner's syndrome. Preganglionic causes include tumors (mediastinal, apical, thyroid), trauma, pneumothorax, cervical infections, brachial plexus syndromes, carotid artery dissection, aneurysm, trauma. Postganglionic causes include neck lesion, head trauma, migraine, cavernous sinus lesion, vascular lesions (carotid dissection, carotid-cavernous fistula, internal carotid artery aneurysm), and infections.

4. How long has he noticed the ptosis? Does it vary? Has he noticed the difference in pupil size? Any change in vision or double vision? Has he had any head or eye trauma? Any pain, headache, or other neurologic symptoms? On exam, what are his visual acuity, pupillary response, and extraocular motility? What does the cranial nerve exam show?

5. This depends on whether the abnormal pupil is smaller (ie, greater anisocoria in a dim/dark room) or larger (ie, greater anisocoria in a bright/light room). For a miotic pupil, the differential diagnosis includes Horner's syndrome, Argyll Robertson pupil, iritis, and pharmacologic (pilocarpine, brimonidine, narcotics, insecticides). For a mydriatic pupil, the differential diagnosis includes Adie's tonic pupil, CN 3 palsy, Hutchinson's pupil, pharmacologic (mydriatic, cycloplegic, cocaine, hallucinogen), iris damage (trauma, ischemia, or surgery (Urrets-Zavalia syndrome)). If the anisocoria is equal in light and dark, then the diagnosis is physiologic anisocoria (difference in pupil size ≤1 mm).

6. Pharmacologic testing for Horner's syndrome consists of two steps:

   1. Topical cocaine 4–10% to determine the presence of Horner's syndrome: if there is increased anisocoria (after 40 minutes), then Horner's syndrome exists (if the pupillary dilation is equal, then the diagnosis is simple anisocoria).

   2. Topical hydroxyamphetamine 1% (Paredrine) to distinguish between preganglionic and postganglionic lesions: if the dilation is equal then the Horner's syndrome is central or preganglionic; if the dilation is asymmetric then the Horner's syndrome is postganglionic.

A 49-year-old woman reports droopy eyelids for the past 6 months and is interested in surgery. She says sometimes she has to raise her lids to keep her eyes open. Her vision seems to be unchanged, but occasionally when driving she notices that the line on the road is double, especially when she looks to her right. She wears bifocal glasses and has no other past ocular history.

1. What is the differential diagnosis of transient diplopia?
2. What additional history would be helpful?

Additional information: the patient is suspected of having myasthenia gravis (MG).

3. What are the characteristic eye findings of this disease and what tests would be useful for confirming the diagnosis?
4. What other workup and treatment are necessary for this disease?

1. The most common causes of transient diplopia are decompensated phoria, convergence or divergence insufficiency, MG, and spasm of accommodation. Other etiologies include GCA (extraocular muscle [EOM] ischemia), vertibrobasilar insufficiency, superior oblique myokymia, cyclic esotropia, and skew deviation.

2. Is the ptosis worse on one side, does it vary (ie, throughout the day, from day to day, when she is tired)? Has she ever had diplopia before? Does it happen with other activities such as reading, watching TV, etc.? Is it associated with a headache or other neurologic symptoms? Has she had any eye or head trauma? Any other medical problems, specifically autoimmune disorders? Any weakness, difficulty in breathing or swallowing, hoarseness?

3. The characteristic ocular findings of MG are asymmetric ptosis and variable strabismus. Gaze-evoked nystagmus also occurs. There is no pupil or ciliary muscle involvement. The hallmark of the disease is variability and fatigability, so there is worsening of the ptosis with extended upgaze and improvement with rest or cold. This can be evaluated with the rest test (improvement in ptosis after closing the eyes for 30 minutes) or ice test (improvement in ptosis after application of an ice pack for 2 minutes). Forced ductions are negative. A Tensilon test can be administered to observe for improvement in ocular signs; however, a negative test does not rule out MG. The diagnostic lab test is acetylcholine (ACh) receptor antibodies. If these tests are negative, then definitive diagnosis is by single fiber electromyography of peripheral or orbicularis muscles.

4. It is important to rule out thyroid disease, thymoma, and other autoimmune disorders, so lab tests (thyroid function tests, ANA, and rheumatoid factor (RF)) and a chest CT or MRI scan should be obtained. The patient should be referred to a neurologist or internist for systemic treatment. Strabismus can be managed with prism spectacles and potentially surgery when stable for at least 6 months.

A 32-year-old woman complains of diplopia for several weeks. She has also had headaches for months. On exam you find an obese, slightly anxious woman with vision of 20/25 in both eyes, normal pupillary response, and esotropia in primary gaze. The optic nerve appearance is shown.

1. What is the abnormality?

2. What is the differential diagnosis?

3. What other tests would you perform in the office?

4. What is the workup for papilledema, and how do you determine whether she has idiopathic intracranial hypertension (IIH)?

Additional information: the patient has IIH.

5. What are the associations?

6. What is the treatment?

7. What is the most likely cause of her diplopia?

1. Bilateral optic disc swelling.

2. Papilledema (intracranial mass, infection, infiltration, hemorrhage, or IIH [pseudotumor cerebri]), malignant hypertension, diabetic papillitis, or compressive optic neuropathy (TRO, IOI).

3. Check the pupils for a RAPD, color vision, visual fields, extraocular motility (consider forced ductions), lid position and presence of proptosis and resistance of the globes to retropulsion. The patient's blood pressure must be checked to rule out hypertension. She should also have a serum blood glucose level.

4. Neuroimaging and lumbar puncture (LP). IIH is a diagnosis of exclusion that is determined by four criteria:

   1. Signs and symptoms of increased intracranial pressure (ie, headache, vomiting, papilledema).

   2. High CSF pressure (>250 mmH$_2$O) with normal composition.

   3. Normal neuroimaging studies.

   4. Normal neurologic examination except for possible CN 6 palsies.

5. IIH is associated with medications (steroids [use or withdrawal], oral contraceptive pills [due to hypercoagulability and dural sinus thrombosis], vitamin A, tetracycline, nalidixic acid, lithium, and isotretinoin), chronic obstructive lung disease, dural sinus thrombosis, radical neck surgery, recent weight gain, and pregnancy.

6. Any medication associated with IIH should be discontinued, and a weight loss regimen should be instituted for obesity. Patients with vision loss, VF defects, or intractable headaches are treated with systemic medications (acetazolamide [Diamox] or furosemide [Lasix]). Patients with progressive visual loss may require surgery (ON sheath fenestration, lumbar-peritoneal shunt).

7. CN 6 palsy.

A 48-year-old man reports being hit by an elbow in his left eye while playing basketball yesterday night. He complains of pain, swelling, and sensitivity to light. Exam of the left eye reveals a visual acuity of 20/40, limited supraduction, and an external exam as noted in the photo. There is subconjunctival hemorrhage and anterior chamber cells and flare. The posterior segment is normal.

1. What would you expect to see on orbital CT scan?
2. What other signs may be present?
3. How would you treat this patient?
4. What are the indications for surgery?
5. If this patient were a child, how would the management differ?

1. The presentation is consistent with an orbital floor fracture with entrapment, which should be evident on orbital CT scan. This is the most common type of orbital fracture, and usually involves the maxillary bone and the posterior medial floor, the weakest point of the orbit.

2. Other signs of a blowout fracture are globe ptosis, infraorbital nerve hypesthesia, and lid emphysema.

3. Initially, the patient should be treated with ice compresses, nasal decongestants, and avoid blowing his nose. Consideration should be given to prescribing oral antibiotics and steroids for 10 days. He also has a traumatic iritis, which should be treated with a topical steroid and cycloplegic. He should be reevaluated for surgery in 7–10 days to allow for reduction of swelling.

4. The indications for repair are diplopia, muscle entrapment, enophthalmos, and facial asymmetry.

5. Pediatric floor fractures are different from those in adults because the bones are pliable and a trapdoor situation may occur, in which the inferior rectus or surrounding tissue can become entrapped. Nausea and bradycardia occur owing to the oculocardiac reflex. This is commonly referred to as a "white-eyed blowout fracture" because the eye is usually quiet; however, it requires emergent surgery to prevent permanent damage to the entrapped tissue.

A 63-year-old man reports difficulty in reading. He says that the words are clear, but he has trouble following the lines of text and loses his place. He denies any change in vision, headaches, or other neurologic symptoms. Exam shows visual acuity of 20/20 in both eyes at distance and near, normal pupillary response without a RAPD, early cataracts, and normal fundus exam.

1. What other tests would you perform?

Additional information: extraocular motility is full and the eyes are orthophoric. Amsler grid reveals a blurry area inferotemporal to fixation in the right eye. Humphrey VF testing shows:

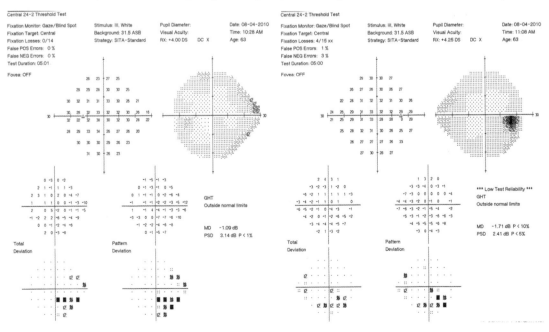

2. What does the VF test show?
3. Where is the pathology?
4. What would you do next?

1. Extraocular motility including alternate cover testing, Amsler grid, and VFs.
2. The visual fields reveal right homonymous inferior quadrantic scotomas.
3. This indicates a lesion involving the left parietal lobe.
4. Obtain neuroimaging, which should be coordinated with the patient's internist.

A 50-year-old man complains of double vision beginning 2 days ago.

1. What do the photos demonstrate?
2. What is the differential diagnosis?
3. What exam findings would be helpful to determine the diagnosis?

Additional information: the patient does have contralateral abducting nystagmus, but no ptosis or other motility limitations.

4. What is the diagnosis?
5. Where is the lesion?
6. What are the etiologies?
7. What are the signs of bilateral involvement?
8. How does this differ from one-and-a-half syndrome?

1. Horizontal gaze palsy with an inability to adduct the left eye.

2. Internuclear ophthalmoplegia, medial rectus palsy, myasthenia gravis.

3. The presence of other neurologic signs, contralateral abducting nystagmus (internuclear ophthalmoplegia [INO]), absence of convergence (anterior INO), absent doll's head maneuvers and caloric stimulation (INO), ptosis (MG), other extraocular motility limitations (MG), variability/fatigability (MG).

4. Internuclear ophthalmoplegia.

5. Medial longitudinal fasciculus (MLF).

6. The etiology depends on age. In patients younger than age 50 years old it is usually demyelination or tumor. In patients older than age 50 years old it is usually vascular. Other causes are trauma, infection, and compression.

7. Inability to adduct either eye, impaired convergence, appearance of exotropia in primary gaze.

8. One-and-a-half syndrome is due to a lesion of the paramedian pontine reticular formation (PPRF) or CN 6 nucleus, and the ipsilateral MLF. This causes ipsilateral gaze palsy and INO, so the only eye movement present is abduction of the contralateral eye with nystagmus. Etiologies include stroke, multiple sclerosis, basilar artery occlusion, and pontine tumors.

A 61-year-old man complains of double vision for the past month.

1. What abnormality is present in the photo?
2. What are the differential diagnosis and most likely diagnosis?

1. Globe dystopia with the left globe displaced inferiorly.

2. Globe dystopia is caused by a mass lesion. The differential diagnosis of adult orbital tumors is large, but the most common tumors are: cavernous hemangioma, meningioma, neurilemmoma, fibrous histiocytoma, lymphoid lesion, lacrimal gland and sinus tumors, and metastases. Patient age, direction of globe displacement, and presence or absence of pain help to narrow the diagnosis. Most lesions are intraconal masses that cause proptosis. Lacrimal and sinus tumors typically cause the globe to be displaced inferiorly. In this case, the patient's left eye is being pushed down and out, which is probably due to a sinus mucocele, most commonly from the frontoethmoid sinus.

Additional information: a CT scan is obtained to confirm the diagnosis.

3. Describe the findings. What is the diagnosis?

4. What is the treatment?

5. If instead the CT scan showed a well-circumscribed fusiform tumor, and the histopathology appeared as in the figure below, what would be the diagnosis?

3. The CT scan shows opacification of the left anterior ethmoid sinus with erosion into the orbit. This represents a sinus mucocele.

4. Surgical excision and IV antibiotics.

5. The figure demonstrates the typical arrangement of spindle cells in an Antoni A-pattern neurilemmoma.

A 46-year-old man complains of poor vision for years. On exam his BSCVA is 20/200 OU, color vision and contrast sensitivity are decreased, the cup-to-disc ratio is normal and there is optic disc pallor OU.

1. What other history would you like to know?

Additional information: the patient reports a gradual deterioration of his vision over the last 6 years but cannot be more specific. Although he suffered several sports related concussions in college, he denies any ocular trauma or eye disease and is unaware of any family history of eye problems except for cataracts. His only medication is a statin for high cholesterol, although he does have a history of taking multiple antibiotics after a positive PPD skin test. He works as a bartender and admits to recreational drug use and struggling with alcohol abuse in the past.

2. What is the differential diagnosis?
3. What testing would you perform?

Additional information: visual field testing shows bilateral central scotomas; MRI of the head and orbits is normal.

4. What diagnosis do you suspect?
5. What are the causes of toxic optic neuropathy?
6. What are the causes of nutritional optic neuropathy?

1. It is important to obtain a complete past medical and ocular history, medication history, family history, and social history, with specific attention to any factors that can contribute to optic nerve damage. Specifically, does the patient have a history of any eye disorders, trauma, surgery, systemic disease with ocular manifestations, malignancy or infectious disease, major blood loss, radiation treatment, or using medications with ocular toxicity? Is there any hereditary eye disease in the family? What are his alcohol, drug, tobacco and nutrition habits? It would also be helpful to know about the timing and progression of the visual loss and how it affected each eye.

2. Optic neuropathy: hereditary, compressive, infiltrative, infectious, toxic, nutritional, traumatic, or retrobulbar.

3. Visual field exam and CT or MRI scan to rule out compressive or infiltrative etiology.

4. Toxic or possibly nutritional optic neuropathy.

5. Ethambutol is the most common; others include isoniazid, rifampin, chloramphenicol, streptomycin, sulfonamides, methanol, arsenic, lead, digitalis, chloroquine, quinine, linezolid, imipramine, cisplatin, busulfan, vincristine, disulfuram, cyclosporine, and tobacco-related or alcohol-related amblyopia. Ischemic-like optic neuropathy can occur with phosphodiesterase 5 inhibitors (sildenafil, vardenafil, tadalafil) and amiodorone.

6. Vitamin deficiencies: B1 (thiamine), B2 (riboflavin), B6 (pyridoxine), B12 (cobalamin), and folic acid.

A 58-year-old woman complains of pain and swelling of her right eye for the past month, with increasing redness over the last week.

1. What is the differential diagnosis?
2. What other history would be helpful?

Additional information: she has double vision but denies any fever, nausea, vomiting or recent trauma or infection. She has hypertension, which is well controlled with an oral medication. She is otherwise healthy and has not had similar symptoms in the past.

3. How would you work up this patient?

Additional information: exam shows restricted extraocular motility with positive forced ductions OD. Palpation of the lids and globes demonstrates fullness of the right upper eyelid laterally and resistance to retropulsion. Proptosis is present by Hertel exophthalmometry. Anterior and posterior segment exams are normal except for conjunctival injection and chemosis. The IOP is normal. Thyroid function tests are normal. CT scan shows an enlarged lacrimal gland and extraocular muscle enlargement with involvement of the tendons.

4. What is the most likely diagnosis?
5. What is the treatment?
6. What is Tolosa–Hunt syndrome?

1. The differential diagnosis for ocular pain, eyelid edema and erythema, and conjunctival injection and chemosis includes: trauma, orbital cellulitis, vasculitis, tumor, arteriovenous fistula, cavernous sinus thrombosis, and thyroid-related ophthalmopathy.

2. Has she noticed a change in vision or double vision? Has she had any ocular trauma or surgery? Any recent infection? Does she have any systemic diseases, particularly autoimmune disorders or cancer? Has she had any previous episodes?

3. Complete eye exam with attention to visual acuity, pupillary response, extraocular motility, proptosis, lid/adnexal masses, cornea (sensation, exposure), intraocular pressure, anterior chamber reaction, and optic nerve appearance (disc edema). Consider thyroid function tests. Orbital CT or MRI scan to rule out mass, abscess, and evaluate muscles/tendons.

4. Idiopathic orbital inflammatory disease (IOI, orbital pseudotumor).

5. Treatment is with high-dose oral steroids (80–100 mg qd for 1 week, then taper over 6 weeks).

6. Tolosa–Hunt syndrome is a form of IOI involving the superior orbital fissure, optic canal, and cavernous sinus causing decreased vision and painful ophthalmoplegia.

A 66-year-old woman complains of increasing droopiness of her eyelids for 20 years. The image demonstrates her appearance in upgaze.

1. What abnormalities are present?
2. What is the differential diagnosis?

Additional information: eye exam shows BSCVA of 20/40 OU, limited extraocular motility in all direction of gaze (even with doll's head maneuvers), absent Bell's phenomenon, negative forced ductions, and fundus appearance as shown:

3. What is the diagnosis?
4. What are the features of this condition?
5. Would you perform any testing?

1. The patient has ptosis (left upper eyelid > right upper eyelid) and inability to elevate eyes (limited extraocular motility).

2. Myasthenia gravis (MG), chronic progressive external ophthalmoplegia (CPEO), myotonic dystrophy, vertical gaze palsy, progressive supranuclear palsy, dorsal midbrain syndrome.

3. CPEO, specifically, Kearns–Sayre syndrome (disorder of mitochondrial DNA [gene deletion impairs oxidative phosphorylation]).

4. Ophthalmoplegia, ptosis, retinal pigment degeneration, and cardiac conduction defects (arrhythmias, heart block, cardiomyopathy); also associated with mental retardation, short stature, deafness, ataxia, and elevated cerebrospinal fluid protein.

5. EKG to detect cardiac abnormalities (patient should have a cardiology consult). Consider muscle biopsy for abnormal "ragged red" fibers or EMG. Tensilon test, ice pack test, or antiACh receptor antibody test can be performed to rule out MG.

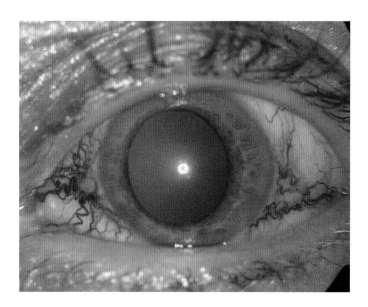

A 62-year-old woman complains that her left eye is red.

1. What notable finding is shown?
2. What is the most likely diagnosis and what is the differential diagnosis?

Additional information: the patient has a history of head trauma, and an MRI shows a dilated superior ophthalmic vein.

3. What is the diagnosis?
4. What other findings can occur?

1. Prominent, dilated, corkscrew scleral and episcleral vessels.

2. This most likely represents an arteriovenous fistula (carotid-cavernous sinus fistula or dural-sinus fistula). Other possibilities are orbital varix, idiopathic orbital inflammatory disease, iritis, or scleritis.

3. Carotid-cavernous sinus fistula.

4. This is a direct, high flow AV communication that can cause a variety of other ocular findings including conjunctival injection and chemosis, elevated IOP, proptosis, orbital bruit, dilated tortuous retinal veins, and, less commonly, CN 6 palsy, anterior segment ischemia, blood in Schlemm's canal, optic nerve cupping, ischemic maculopathy, and retinal artery occlusion.

1. What abnormality of the optic nerve is shown?
2. What is the pathophysiology of this disorder?
3. Are there any associations?
4. What is the prognosis?
5. What are other optic nerve dysplasias?

1. Optic nerve coloboma demonstrating a dysplastic nerve head with large abnormal appearing disc elongated inferiorly with an irregular vascular pattern.

2. Incomplete closure of the embryonic fissure results in clefts of ocular structures, usually located inferonasally, and can be unilateral or bilateral.

3. Optic nerve colobomas are associated with other ocular colobomas (ie, eyelid, iris, ciliary body, choroid, retina), and they may also be associated with systemic abnormalities such as congenital heart defects, double aortic arch, coarctation of the aorta, transposition of the great vessels, intracranial carotid anomalies, and basal encephalocele.

4. Optic nerve coloboma causes variable but nonprogressive visual acuity and visual field defects depending on the severity of the nerve involvement, which can be severe (complete chorioretinal coloboma) to mild (slight optic nerve deformity resembling physiologic cupping).

5. Other types of optic nerve dysplasias include hypoplasia, morning glory syndrome (may represent a form of coloboma), optic nerve drusen, pit, and tilted optic disc.

A mother brings in her 5-month-old boy because his eyes have been tearing for a couple of months. On further questioning, she reports no discharge or redness, but he squints and turns away from bright lights. He has no significant past ocular or medical history.

1. What is the differential diagnosis?
2. What exam findings would you look for?

Additional information: retinoscopy shows a refractive error of –1.00 D OU, vision is CSM (central, steady, maintain) OU, anterior segment appearance is similar to that shown in the photo, and posterior segment exam shows a cup-to-disc ratio of 0.5 OU.

3. What finding is depicted and what is the diagnosis?
4. What would you tell the mother about the diagnosis?
5. What is the treatment?

1. Possible diagnoses include nasolacrimal duct obstruction (NLDO), corneal abrasion, foreign body, iritis, and congenital glaucoma.

2. Specific signs to look for on exam include increased lacrimal lake, discharge from lacrimal puncta, corneal staining, foreign body on the ocular surface or tarsal conjunctiva, anterior chamber cell and flare, buphthalmos, myopia, enlarged corneas, increased IOP, and optic disc cupping.

3. Haab's striae (breaks in Descemet's membrane), which is a sign of congenital glaucoma.

4. Congenital glaucoma occurs in the first few months of life, is usually bilateral, and can be primary (developmental abnormality of the angle structures, most commonly due to a mutation in the *CYP1B1* gene), secondary, or associated with ocular or systemic syndromes. An examination under anesthesia may be required to check tonometry, corneal diameter, gonioscopy, and ophthalmoscopy.

5. Treatment is surgical. Topical medications (beta-blockers or carbonic anhydrase inhibitors) are used to control IOP until surgery can be performed. Brimonidine is contraindicated because it can be associated with death. Surgical options include goniotomy (children <1.5 years old with clear cornea) and trabeculotomy (cloudy cornea, children >1.5 years old, or two failed goniotomies). If these fail, then trabeculectomy with mitomycin C, glaucoma drainage implant, and cycloablation are options. Correction of any refractive error and treatment of amblyopia must also be performed.

A 6-month-old girl is noted to have a watery eye. The mother says sometimes the lashes are crusty, especially in the inner corner.

1. What additional history would you ask the mother?
2. What other finding would you look for on exam, and what other tests may be helpful?

Additional information: the eye has been watery for 1 month, no redness or discharge has been noted, and there does not seem to be any irritation. The baby has not been treated and has not been sick or around anyone with a cold or eye infection. Palpation of the lacrimal sac produces some scant mucus reflux from the punctum, and dye disappearance test shows delayed clearance of fluorescein from the tear film. The other tests could not be performed.

3. What is the most likely diagnosis and its usual etiology?
4. How would you treat the baby?

1. Is there any redness, itching, or discharge? How long have the symptoms been present? Has this ever happened before? Has any treatment been initiated? Has the baby recently had a cold or contact with someone with a cold or eye infection? Is there any past medical history?

2. Mucoid reflux with digital pressure over the lacrimal sac and conjunctivitis. Dye disappearance test, Jones I and II tests, and nasolacrimal irrigation.

3. Congenital nasolacrimal duct obstruction, which is usually due to a membrane covering the valve of Hasner.

4. Treatment consists of lacrimal sac massage and compresses. Antibiotic drops can be used, especially when there is crusting. If the condition does not resolve spontaneously, then nasolacrimal duct probing should be performed by 13 months of age.

You are asked to see a 3-year-old girl with an eye turn. Apparently the child's eyes have turned inward since she was a baby, but now the mother notices that the left eye also goes up.

1. What is the differential diagnosis?
2. What exam findings would enable you to determine the correct diagnosis?

Additional information: her best-corrected visual acuity is 20/20 OU with +1.00 D OD and +1.50 D OS. The AC/A ratio is normal. The ET is comitant and measures 35 prism diopters at distance and near. She does cross fixate, and there is inferior oblique overaction but no V pattern. There is also no dissociated vertical deviation (DVD) or latent nystagmus present. Worth 4 dot testing demonstrates suppression OS. There is also a history of strabismus in the father. Anterior and posterior segment exams are normal.

3. What type of esotropia does this girl have?
4. How would you treat her?
5. If this child also had a DVD, what surgical procedures could be used to correct it?

Additional information: on postoperative day one following strabismus surgery, a large exotropia is noted and there is no adduction of the left eye.

6. What is the diagnosis and treatment?

1. The esotropia (ET) may be congenital, accommodative, nonaccommodative, mixed, or due to Duane's syndrome (type 1) or a congenital CN 6 palsy.

2. It is important to know the visual acuity and whether there is any amblyopia or refractive error. What is the AC/A ratio? The ocular motility must be assessed and the deviation measured at distance and near. Is the deviation comitant or incomitant, is there an A or V pattern, and is there any oblique muscle overaction? Does she have a DVD? Is there latent nystagmus? Does she cross fixate? Is there a suppression scotoma?

3. Congenital ET.

4. Rule out an accommodative component by prescribing glasses with the full cycloplegic refraction. Strabismus surgery is performed on either one eye with a medial rectus recession and lateral rectus resection (R&R), or both eyes with bilateral medial rectus recessions. The inferior oblique overaction is also treated surgically with a weakening procedure.

5. Bilateral superior rectus recession, inferior rectus resection, or inferior oblique weakening or anterior transposition.

6. Lost medial rectus muscle after ET repair, which requires return to the operating room to find the muscle and reattach it to the globe, making sure to use locking bites to prevent a slipped muscle.

A 3-year-old boy is brought to your office because his eyes jiggle. Exam shows horizontal oscillations of the eyes.

1. What is the differential diagnosis?

2. The boy turns his head to the side. If the nystagmus dampens in right gaze, what direction is the boy's head turn?

3. What are the typical features of motor nystagmus?

4. What treatments can be used for congenital nystagmus?

5. What is the triad of findings in spasmus nutans?

6. What is the work up of spasmus nutans?

1. Congenital nystagmus is most commonly afferent (due to sensory deprivation), efferent (motor), latent, or spasmus nutans. It is important to rule out acquired nystagmus.

2. Left head turn to place the eyes in the direction of the null point.

3. The characteristics of motor nystagmus are: usually horizontal in all positions of gaze, increased intensity with fixation, presence of a null point, decreased by convergence, absent during sleep, may have latent component, reversal with horizontal optokinetic nystagmus (OKN) testing, and associated strabismus.

4. Consider base-out prism glasses to stimulate convergence and thereby dampen the nystagmus. If there is a head turn >50% of the time to keep eyes in null point, then surgical correction with the Kestenbaum procedure can be performed.

5. Fine, rapid, asymmetric eye movements, head nodding, and torticollis.

6. Spasmus nutans is a diagnosis of exclusion, so a careful exam of the pupils (RAPD) and optic nerve is necessary, and neuroimaging is indicated to rule out a tumor (chiasmal glioma or parasellar tumor, which can produce similar eye movements). Spasmus nutans is benign and disappears by the age of 5 years.

This child's mother brings him in for a routine eye exam. There is no past ocular history.

1. What abnormality does this patient have?

2. What are the associated eye disorders?

3. What are your recommendations for eye care?

1. Down syndrome.

2. Refractive errors (most commonly hyperopia), strabismus, nystagmus, amblyopia, lid abnormalities (epicanthal folds, upward slanting of palpebral fissures, blepharitis, chalazia, NLDO), keratoconus, iris Brushfield spots, cataracts, glaucoma.

3. The patient should have routine eye exams to monitor for associated ocular disorders. Any refractive error should be corrected and amblyopia treatment should be instituted if necessary. Strabismus, blepharitis, keratoconus, cataracts, and glaucoma may also require treatment.

A 16-year-old boy complains of double vision for the last 4 days. He denies any blurry or decreased vision. You notice that he tilts his head to the side, and he says he does this to makes the double disappear. On exam, his vision is 20/20 in both eyes, pupillary response is normal, ocular motility shows a left hypertropia. The rest of the exam is normal.

1. What test would you perform to diagnose the problem?

Additional information: he has a left hypertropia that is worse in right gaze and with left head tilt.

2. What is the diagnosis and what other history would be relevant?
3. What head position would the boy have?
4. The patient plays football and says he was stunned after a rough tackle. How would you treat him?

1. Parks–Bielschowsky 3-step test. If this shows a superior oblique palsy, then vertical fusion amplitudes would be helpful to distinguish between congenital and other causes.

2. Left superior oblique palsy, which is most commonly congenital or traumatic. This could be a decompensated congenital superior oblique (SO) palsy or a traumatic one. It would be helpful to ask about recent illness or trauma. It is also necessary to ask about other neurologic symptoms. Old photographs may be useful to determine whether there was a long-standing head posture.

3. The head is positioned in the direction of action of the weak muscle in order to minimize the diplopia. Therefore he would have his chin down, face turned to the opposite side, and head tilted to the opposite shoulder.

4. For an isolated palsy, the initial treatment is observation and prism glasses or occlusion of one eye to alleviate the diplopia. If there are other neurologic deficits, then neuroimaging is indicated. The palsy may improve with time. If it does not and is stable for at least 6 months, then muscle surgery can be considered. The Knapp classification is helpful for determining the best procedure. The Harado Ito procedure (lateral transposition of superior oblique tendon) may be used to correct the torsional component.

A 6-year-old girl is noted to have an eye turn. Her extraocular motility is demonstrated in the photos.

1. What is the diagnosis?

2. What is the appropriate treatment?

3. Does this child demonstrate oblique muscle overaction?

1. V-pattern exotropia (XT).

2. Correct any refractive error and treat amblyopia if present. The XT can be treated with overminused spectacles to induce accommodative convergence, fusional convergence training with progressive base-out prism, or prism therapy with base-in prisms. If the ocular misalignment is present >50% of the time, then surgery is necessary. A prism adaptation test is performed to uncover the full amount of deviation. Surgical correction is performed on either one eye with a lateral rectus recession and medial rectus resection (R&R), or both eyes with bilateral lateral rectus recessions. The V pattern is corrected with horizontal rectus muscle transposition (in the direction of the desired weakening [mnemonic: MALE – Medial recti moved toward Apex of pattern or Lateral recti moved toward Empty space of pattern]) or with oblique muscle weakening, depending on whether or not there is any oblique overaction.

3. Yes, the photos show bilateral inferior oblique overaction.

You are called to the ER to see a 7-month-old boy because his right eye turns in and he has a funny red reflex. Exam shows poor fixation with the right eye and ability to fix and follow with the left eye. Anterior segment appears normal in both eyes. There is a dim red reflex in the right eye and a normal red reflex in the left eye. Dilated fundus exam shows vitreous hemorrhage in the right eye and intraretinal hemorrhages in both eyes.

1. What is the differential diagnosis?
2. What questions would you ask the parents?

Additional information: the mother says she noticed the eye turn for 1 week. Her pregnancy was uneventful and the birth was uncomplicated. The baby was full term, normal weight, and did not require supplemental oxygen. There is no past medical history and no known trauma.

3. How would you work up and treat this patient?

1. Shaken baby syndrome, trauma, retinopathy of prematurity.

2. How long have the findings been present? What is the birth history (premature, low birth weight, supplemental oxygen)? Is there any other medical history? Is there any history of trauma? How is the baby developing, sleeping, eating? What is the situation at home? Is the baby difficult/crying/colicky?

3. Radiology studies (CT scan and/or plain films) to rule out other traumatic injuries. Report case to child protective services and authorities for suspected shaken baby syndrome. The baby must be monitored for amblyopia OD and may require vitrectomy for nonclearing vitreous hemorrhage. He should also have a pediatric consultation and may require treatment of other injuries.

A 9-month-old girl has a puffy, red, blotchy, left upper eyelid that has been present since shortly after birth.

1. What is the diagnosis?
2. What are the potential ocular complications of this lesion?
3. What are the most important parts of the eye exam to check?
4. What are the treatment options?
5. What systemic syndrome is associated with this tumor?

1. Capillary hemangioma, which is the most common benign eyelid tumor in children.

2. Eyelid capillary hemangiomas may cause ptosis or astigmatism resulting in anisometropia, strabismus, or amblyopia.

3. It is important to determine whether the lid lesion is affecting vision. Therefore it is critical to measure the visual acuity, refractive error, ocular alignment, and motility.

4. Treat any refractive error and amblyopia if present. Most capillary hemangiomas regress by age 10 years old; however, if the tumor is affecting vision it may require intervention with intralesional (risk of central retinal artery occlusion) or systemic steroids, systemic propranolol, laser photocoagulation, embolization, or excision. Topical timolol may also be effective and is a safer alternative to the aforementioned traditional treatments.

5. Kassabach–Merritt syndrome, which is a consumptive coagulopathy with platelet trapping that causes thrombocytopenia and cardiac failure and has a mortality rate of 30%.

A mother brings her 2-year-old daughter to see you because she notices the girl's pupils look funny in certain lighting conditions. The child has normal vision and ocular motility. Slit lamp exam reveals the abnormality seen in the photo.

1. What is the diagnosis?

2. What is the etiology of bilateral congenital cataracts?

3. What is the treatment?

4. When a patient with the type of cataract shown above undergoes phacoemulsification, there is an increased risk of what complication?

5. What routine step of cataract surgery should not be performed?

1. Posterior polar cataract.

2. Idiopathic, hereditary (usually autosomal dominant [AD]), metabolic, associated with ocular disorder, intrauterine infection (TORCH – [Toxoplasma, Other viruses, Rubella, Cytomegalovirus, Herpesvirus]), maternal drug ingestion or malnutrition, or trauma.

3. The treatment depends on the size of the cataract and whether it is affecting vision. The critical size for causing vision impairment is ≥3 mm. Posterior polar cataracts <3 mm in diameter should be followed closely for growth and decreased visual acuity. Surgery (cataract extraction and IOL insertion) is performed when the cataract is visually significant.

4. Posterior capsular rupture with possible vitreous loss and/or retained lens material.

5. A posterior capsular defect is often present, so hydrodissection should not be performed since this step can rupture the posterior capsule. Also, polishing/vacuuming the central posterior capsule of residual lens material/plaque should be avoided because even gentle manipulation of this area can cause a break in the posterior capsule. Any remaining opacity can be safely removed with a primary posterior capsulorhexis at the time of surgery or a Nd:YAG laser capsulotomy at a later date.

You are called to the neonatal intensive care unit (NICU) to see a 31-week-old premature infant. The retinal appearance is demonstrated in the photo.

1. What is the diagnosis?
2. What is the classification system of this disorder?
3. What are the risk factors?
4. What is plus disease?
5. When is treatment indicated?

Additional information: retinal exam reveals this baby's disease is Zone 2, Stage 3, without Plus disease.

6. How would you treat him?
7. What is the prognosis?
8. What are the potential complications?

1. Stage 3 retinopathy of prematurity (ROP).

2. ROP is classified by the type of retinal changes (stage), location (zone), and clock hours of retinal involvement (extent):

   Stage 1 = flat, circumferential, thin, white, demarcation line between the posterior vascularized and peripheral avascular retina.

   Stage 2 = demarcation line becomes elevated and organized into a pink-white ridge, no fibrovascular growth visible.

   Stage 3 = extraretinal fibrovascular proliferation from the surface of the ridge.

   Stage 4 = dragging of vessels and subtotal traction retinal detachment:
   - 4A = macula attached
   - 4B = macula detached.

   Stage 5 = total retinal detachment.

   Zone 1 = inner zone (posterior pole) corresponding to the area enclosed by a circle around the optic disc with a radius equal to twice the distance from the disc to the macula (diameter of 60 degrees).

   Zone 2 = the area between Zone 1 and a circle centered on the optic disc and tangent to the nasal ora serrata.

   Zone 3 = the remaining temporal crescent of retina (last area to become vascularized).

3. Premature birth (<33 weeks' gestation), low birth weight (<1.5 kg), supplemental oxygen (>50 days) and complicated hospital course. The risk of ROP increases exponentially with earlier prematurity and lower birth weight since at 36 weeks the nasal retina is completely vascularized; at 40 weeks, temporal retina is fully vascularized.

4. Plus disease occurs when there are at least two quadrants of shunted blood, which produces engorged, tortuous vessels in the posterior pole, vitreous haze, and iris vascular congestion. This is a poor prognostic sign. Aggressive posterior (AP) ROP or Rush disease is plus disease in Zone 1 or posterior Zone 2, which is usually rapidly progressive.

5. Treatment indicated for threshold disease (ie, Stage 3 + disease with at least 5 contiguous or 8 noncontiguous clock hours of involvement in Zone 1 or 2), which represents the level at which 50% will go blind without treatment.

   The Early Treatment of ROP (ETROP) Study concluded that ablation of peripheral avascular retina with laser photocoagulation should be performed earlier (ie, type 1 ROP, which is defined as: Zone 1, any stage of ROP with Plus disease; Zone 1, Stage 3 with or without Plus disease; Zone 2, Stage 2 or 3 with Plus disease). The Cryo-ROP study showed that ablation with cryotherapy for Zone 1 disease was beneficial. The BEAT-ROP Study showed that intravitreal injection of bevacizumab for Zone 1 disease was beneficial, but long-term safety has not been studied. For Stage 4 or greater, pars plana vitrectomy is recommended.

6. This baby does not require treatment. He should have serial retinal exams every 1–2 weeks until the extreme retinal periphery is vascularized, then monthly exams.

7. The prognosis depends on the amount and stage of ROP. Up to 90% of cases resolve spontaneously.

8. High myopia, strabismus, amblyopia, macular dragging, nystagmus, glaucoma, cataracts, keratoconus, band keratopathy, retinal detachment, and phthisis bulbi.

An 8-year-old girl complains of headaches in school. On exam her uncorrected vision is 20/30 OD and 20/25 OS, manifest refraction of +1.00 D OD and –1.00 D OS yields 20/30 OD and 20/15 OS. Anterior and posterior segment exams are normal.

1. What is the next test you would perform?

Additional information: cycloplegic refraction reveals +4.00 D OD and +1.00 D OS with vision of 20/30 and 20/20, respectively.

2. What is the diagnosis?
3. How would you manage this patient?
4. What are the levels of anisometropia (myopic, hyperopic, and astigmatic) that require correction to prevent possible amblyopia?
5. What are the types of amblyopia?

1. Cycloplegic refraction.

2. Hyperopia and anisometropic amblyopia OD.

3. She should be prescribed the full cycloplegic refraction and patching/penalization therapy started OS for no more than 1 week per year of age before re-examination. This is continued until the vision in the right eye has normalized or stabilized.

   In an older patient who may not tolerate the full prescription, a postcycloplegic refraction pushing plus is necessary and the glasses prescription may need to be increased gradually over time. If the patient is unable to adapt to the degree of anisometropia in the glasses, then consider treatment with a contact lens or laser vision correction OD.

4. Myopic anisometropia $\geq$3 D, hyperopic anisometropia $\geq$1 D, and astigmatic anisometropia $\geq$1.5 D.

5. Strabismic, refractive, and deprivation.

This 7-year-old girl was diagnosed with accommodative esotropia (ET). Her mother would like a second opinion and brings her to see you.

1. What are the different types of accommodative ET?
2. How would you measure her AC/A ratio?

Additional information: her vision is 20/20 OD and 20/40 OS with a refractive error of +4.00 D OD and +5.25 D OS, she has an AC/A ratio of 5:1, and measurement of her ET shows similar amounts of deviation at distance and near.

3. What type of ET does she have?
4. How would you treat her?

1. Refractive accommodative (normal AC/A ratio), nonrefractive accommodative (high AC/A ratio), mixed mechanism, and decompensated accommodative.

2. There are 2 methods for determining the AC/A ratio:

   Heterophoria method: AC/A = IPD + [(N−D)/diopter]

   IPD = interpupillary distance (cm); N = near deviation; D = distance deviation; diopter = accommodative demand at fixation distance.

   Lens gradient method: AC/A = (WL−NL)/D

   WL = deviation with lens in front of eye; NL = deviation without lens in front of eye; D = dioptric power of lens used.

3. The high hyperopia, normal AC/A ratio, and similar ET at distance and near indicate that she has a refractive accommodative ET.

4. She should be prescribed the full cycloplegic refraction. The amblyopia OS should be treated with patching or penalization OD for no more than 1 week per year of age before re-examination. Once the vision in the left eye has normalized or stabilized, surgery can be performed for any residual or nonaccommodative component of ET (any deviation >10 PD that is not eliminated with glasses).

A 4-year-old boy is brought to your office because of a droopy eyelid. His mother states that his right eye has always looked smaller.

1. What are the diagnosis and possible etiologies?

2. What would you look for on exam to determine the etiology?

3. What are the characteristic findings of congenital myogenic ptosis?

4. What is the treatment of congenital myogenic ptosis?

5. What is the prognosis?

1. Congenital ptosis, which can be myogenic (most common), neurogenic (congenital CN 3 palsy or Horner's syndrome), or rarely aponeurotic (birth trauma).

2. Visual acuity, levator function, pupil size and response, ocular motility, presence of jaw winking, and iris color.

3. Poor levator function, loss of the lid crease, eyelid lag, sometimes lagophthalmos, and rarely amblyopia.

4. Treat amblyopia if present, then surgical lid repair. For poor levator function, the usual technique is frontalis suspension with silicone rods, fascia lata, or frontalis flap. Maximal levator resection may be useful in some cases.

5. The outcome for congenital ptosis repair is variable and depends on the degree of levator function, poor function being more difficult to treat.

A 23-year-old graduate student says she has a white spot on her eye that she wants removed.

1. What is the diagnosis?
2. What type of tumor is this?
3. Are there any associations?
4. What is the treatment?

1. Limbal dermoid.

2. Choristoma that represents normal tissue in an abnormal location.

3. Limbal dermoids can cause astigmatism and amblyopia. They can be isolated or associated with Goldenhar's syndrome (preauricular skin tags, aural fistulas, eyelid coloboma, and vertebral anomalies).

4. Treatment is observation or surgical excision. When excising a dermoid, it is important to pay particular attention to the depth of the keratectomy to avoid penetration of the globe. A variable amount of corneal scarring may remain.

A 51-year-old man complains of a gradual decrease in vision over years. He states that his vision in the left eye has always been worse than in the right eye, and he has worn glasses since childhood for nearsightedness and astigmatism. He has early cataracts that are similar in both eyes with a best-corrected visual acuity of 20/25 OD and 20/80 OS.

1. What anterior segment findings are evident in the photo?
2. What other questions would you ask this patient?

Additional information: his history is negative except for a complicated delivery at birth.

3. What is the corneal diagnosis and etiology?
4. How is this differentiated from congenital glaucoma?
5. What is the differential diagnosis of a congenital cloudy cornea?
6. What are the treatment options for this patient?

1. Corneal scars and cataract.

2. Is there any history of eye trauma or surgery? Is there a family history of eye disease? What is his past medical history including birth history (ie, birth trauma)?

3. Corneal edema and scarring from Descemet's membrane tears secondary to birth trauma (ie, forceps injury).

4. The breaks in Descemet's membrane from forceps injury are vertical or oblique whereas those from congenital glaucoma (Haab's striae) are oriented horizontally or concentric to the limbus.

5. Mnemonic STUMPED: **S**clerocornea, **T**ear in **D**escemet's membrane, **U**lcers, **M**etabolic disease, **P**eter's anomaly, **E**dema (CHED), **D**ermoid.

   Other causes include congenital hereditary stromal dystrophy (CHSD), rubella, posterior keratoconus, and corneal staphyloma.

6. Corneal transplant with endothelial keratoplasty (DSAEK, DMEK) or penetrating keratoplasty for corneal decompensation.

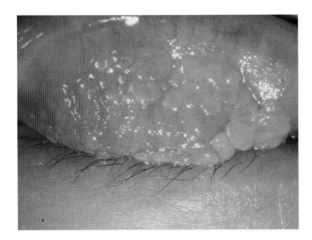

An 11-year-old boy says his eyes have been red and itchy for 2 months. He denies any change in vision but occasionally has some discharge. He has tried Visine with minimal relief. His past ocular and medical history are negative.

1. What is the diagnosis?
2. What is the differential diagnosis, and what are the distinguishing findings?

Additional information: anterior segment exam also reveals this finding:

3. What is the finding, and what is the diagnosis?
4. What other characteristic findings may occur?
5. What is the treatment?
6. What are the possible complications?
7. What is the prognosis?

1. Allergic conjunctivitis.

2. Seasonal or perennial allergic conjunctivitis, giant papillary conjunctivitis, vernal keratoconjunctivitis, and atopic keratoconjunctivitis. GPC, VKC, and AKC are more severe conditions with characteristic findings (ie, large or giant papillae [GPC and VKC], and may have symblepharon [AKC] or keratitis). The age of onset, duration, precipitating factors, associated contact lens wear, and a history of atopy are all helpful in determining the exact diagnosis.

3. The picture shows a Horner–Trantas dot (collection of eosinophils at the limbus). The diagnosis is VKC.

4. Ropy discharge, limbal follicles, and shield ulcer.

5. Chronic therapy with topical steroids and a combination mast cell stabilizer/antihistamine. A steroid with less risk of causing increased IOP and cataract, such as loteprednol, is preferred since patients are young and often require treatment for months or years. The steroids should be tapered slowly and discontinued when possible. Topical cyclosporine may be helpful, as may tacrolimus.

6. Corneal ulceration, scarring, and neovascularization. Steroid treatment can cause cataracts (posterior subcapsular) and increased IOP (and possibly glaucoma).

7. VKC is self-limited. It usually lasts up to 10 years and then resolves. The prognosis is very good if complications do not occur.

A 20-year-old man presents with progressively decreased vision and similar retinal findings in both eyes.

1. What does the picture show?
2. What is the differential diagnosis?
3. What other test may be useful to determine the correct diagnosis?

Additional information: a fluorescein angiogram (FA) is performed.

4. What does the FA show, and what is the diagnosis?
5. How would you treat this patient?
6. What would you tell this patient about the genetics of this disease?
7. What is the prognosis?

1. Deep, symmetric, yellow pisciform (fish-tail shaped) flecks (yellow flecks are groups of enlarged retinal pigment epithelium (RPE) cells packed with a granular substance with ultrastructural, autofluorescent, and histochemical properties consistent with lipofuscin) scattered throughout the posterior pole at the level of the RPE. There is also a "bull's eye" atrophic maculopathy with "beaten bronze" appearance.

2. The pisciform lesions with "bull's eye" maculopathy is most consistent with Stargardt disease, but other causes of a bull's eye include pericentral retinitis pigmentosa, cone and cone-rod dystrophy, age-related macular degeneration (ARMD), central areolar choroidal dystrophy, chloroquine/hydroxychloroquine retinal toxicity, chronic macular hole, olivopontocerebellar atrophy, and ceroid lipofuscinosis.

3. A fluorescein angiogram can highlight the RPE abnormalities of the "bull's eye" maculopathy, but more importantly shows the generalized decreased choroidal fluorescence (dark choroid sign) and a central zone of hyperfluorescence as well as blotchy hyperfluorescent spots that do not correspond to the flecks seen clinically (note: flecks demonstrate early blockage and late hyperfluorescent staining) of Stargardt disease. The flecks appear hyperautofluorescent on fundus autofluorescence imaging due to the excessive lipofuscin deposition; can also show hypoautofluorescence in areas of RPE damage. Optical coherence tomography shows patchy loss of photoreceptor layers corresponding to macular atrophic areas. Color vision is abnormal. Genetic testing with the ABCR400 microarray can find the common ABCA4 polymorphisms with a detection rate of 60–70%.

4. Dark choroid consistent with Stargardt disease.

5. There is no effective treatment. Vitamin A supplementation should be avoided. Low-vision aids would be beneficial.

6. Stargardt disease has been mapped to a mutation in the *STGD1/ABCA4* gene on chromosome 1p21–p22 in the more common autosomal recessive form. In contrast, the autosomal dominant form has been mapped to *STGD4* on chromosome 4p and *STGD3/ELOVL4* on chromosome 6q14 encoding a photoreceptor-specific component of a polyunsaturated fatty acid elongation system. Fundus flavimaculatus has been mapped to *ABCA4* gene on chromosome 1p21–p13.

7. Stargardt disease carries a poor prognosis with vision deteriorating to 20/200 or worse by the 3rd decade of life. The autosomal dominant form has a more benign course with milder color and night vision changes, later onset, and less severe clinical course.

A mother brings her 2-year-old son to see you because she noticed that a recent indoor flash photo showed "red eye" in only one eye. She says it was present in the right eye, but the pupil appeared white in the left eye. On exam the visual acuity is reduced in the left eye, there is a small esotropia, and leukocoria is present.

1. What is the differential diagnosis?

Additional information: there is no family history of eye disease. The boy has a positive RAPD OS and fundus exam shows the following lesion.

2. What is the diagnosis?
3. How would you work up this child?
4. What are the genetics?
5. What is the chance of a sibling having this disorder?
6. What are the characteristic histopathology findings?

1. The differential diagnosis of leukocoria includes cataract, retinoblastoma (RB), retinopathy of prematurity (ROP), and Coats disease. Other etiologies are persistent hyperplastic primary vitreous (PHPV), familial exudative vitreoretinopathy (FEVR), toxocariasis, toxoplasmosis, coloboma, myelinated nerve fibers, retinal detachment, and rarer causes such as retinal dysplasia, cyclitic membrane, incontinentia pigmenti, Norrie disease, retinoschisis, and medulloepithelioma.

2. Retinoblastoma.

3. Neuroimaging is performed to diagnose extraocular extension and trilateral retinoblastoma (bilateral RB with pineal blastoma or parasellar mass). This boy requires an oncology consultation for systemic workup including a bone scan, bone marrow aspirate, and lumbar puncture (cytology).

4. RB has been mapped to chromosome 13q14, and the gene mutation must be present on both chromosomes. RB is 94% sporadic (25% germinal, 75% somatic) and 6% familial (autosomal dominant with 80% penetrance, therefore only 40% manifest a tumor). Most cases occur sporadically in babies with no family history and are unilateral and unifocal. Bilateral cases are typically familial.

5. If there is one affected child, then the risk of a sibling having RB is 1%. (The one affected child is probably a sporadic case and there is only a 6% chance that it is familial. If it is familial, then the risk of another child having RB is 40%.) If there are two affected children, then the risk of a sibling having RB is 40% (this represents familial cases).

6. There are three characteristic histopathology findings of RB:

   Homer–Wright rosette: appears as nuclei surrounding a tangle of neural filaments without a lumen. This represents low-grade neuroblastic differentiation and can also be found in other types of neuroblastic tumors, such as adrenal neuroblastoma and medulloblastoma.

   Flexner–Wintersteiner rosette: appears as a single row of columnar cells in a ring around a central lumen. This represents early retinal differentiation (ie, attempt of outer photoreceptor production) and is also present in medulloepithelioma.

   Fleurette: appears as a bouquet of neoplastic photoreceptor inner segments. This represents the highest degree of photoreceptor differentiation in RB.

7. What pathologic finding is shown below?

8. What are the treatment options?

9. What is the prognosis?

10. What is the Reese–Ellsworth classification?

7. Homer–Wright rosettes.

8. Treatment modalities include enucleation, cryotherapy, laser photocoagulation, external beam radiation, brachytherapy, intraarterial chemotherapy and systemic chemotherapy.

Enucleation is performed on all blind and painful eyes, on the affected eye in most unilateral cases, on the worse eye in most asymmetric cases, and on both eyes in many symmetric cases.

Photocoagulation/cryotherapy is performed occasionally on eyes with one or a few small tumors that do not involve the optic nerve or macula.

External beam radiation is performed on salvageable eyes with vitreous seeding or a large tumor, on most eyes with multifocal tumors, and on eyes that have failed photocoagulation therapy.

Brachytherapy is performed on salvageable eyes with a single medium-sized tumor that does not involve the optic nerve or macula, even with localized vitreous seeding.

Chemoreduction is when systemic chemotherapy is combined with local therapy and is used in globe salvaging management. Chemotherapy delivered by catheters in the ophthalmic artery or carotid artery have been described.

9. The prognosis is generally good: 90–95% survival rate and 3% regress spontaneously.

The prognosis is poor for optic nerve or uveal invasion, extraocular extension, multifocal tumors, or delay in diagnosis. Bilateral RB, degree of necrosis, and calcification do not affect the prognosis. In bilateral cases, the prognosis depends on the status of the tumor in the worse eye.

RB is fatal within 4 years if left untreated. When metastases occur, they are most commonly to the CNS along the optic nerve, and 50% are to bone.

10. The Reese–Ellsworth classification predicts the visual prognosis (not survival) in eyes undergoing radiation treatment. A newer classification system called the International Classification of Retinoblastoma (ICRB) was developed to better predict outcomes:

Group A: Small intraretinal tumors (<3 mm) away from foveola and disc.

Group B: Tumors >3 mm, macular or juxtapapillary location, or with subretinal fluid.

Group C: Tumor with focal subretinal or vitreous seeding within 3 mm of tumor.

Group D: Tumor with diffuse subretinal or vitreous seeding >3 mm from tumor.

Group E: Extensive retinoblastoma occupying >50% of the globe with or without neovascular glaucoma, hemorrhage, extension of tumor to optic nerve or anterior chamber.

A 7-year-old boy complains of double vision. He has no history of trauma. His past medical and family history are negative.

1. What is the differential diagnosis?
2. What additional history would be helpful?
3. What testing would you perform?

1. The patient's diplopia is due to globe displacement, most likely from orbital cellulitis or an orbital mass. Orbital tumors in children are usually benign (90%). The most common lesions are capillary hemangioma, dermoid cyst, and lymphangioma. Other benign lesions include neurofibroma, meningioma, and inflammatory pseudotumor. The differential diagnosis of malignant tumors includes rhabdomyosarcoma, neuroblastoma, teratoma, optic nerve glioma, histiocytic tumors, granulocytic sarcoma, and Burkitt's lymphoma.

2. Is there any pain, redness, or eyelid swelling? Has he had a recent infection or fever? Is there any change in vision? What is the time course of the proptosis?

3. In addition to a comprehensive eye exam with attention to visual acuity, extraocular motility, pupillary reaction, and fundus exam, orbital imaging is necessary.

Additional information: a CT scan and biopsy show:

4. What is the diagnosis?

5. What are the histologic types of this tumor and their characteristics?

6. How would you treat this patient?

7. What is the prognosis?

4. Rhabdomyosarcoma.

5. Embryonal is the most common type and usually occurs in children.

   Botryoid is a rare subtype of embryonal, which can occur in the anterior orbit.

   Alveolar is the second most common, has the worst prognosis, is usually found in the inferior orbit, and often arises in the extremities during adolescence.

   Pleomorphic is the least common type, is the most differentiated, has the best prognosis, and usually occurs in adults.

6. He requires emergent diagnostic biopsy with immunohistochemical staining and a pediatric oncology consultation for systemic workup (abdominal and thoracic CT scan, bone marrow biopsy, and lumbar puncture). Treatment is with a combination of surgery, chemotherapy, and radiation depending on the location and extent of the tumor.

7. The prognosis also depends on the type and extent of the malignancy. With chemotherapy and radiation, the 3-year survival rate is 90%. For localized orbital tumors, the survival rate is up to 95%, but decreases to 60% if there is invasion of adjacent structures.

A 9-year-old girl has unilateral decreased vision and photophobia.

1. What does the photo show?
2. What is the differential diagnosis?

Additional information: the patient's family adopted a puppy 1 month ago.

3. What is the most likely diagnosis?
4. What are the clinical presentations of this disease?
5. What is the causative organism and describe its lifecycle?
6. How is this condition treated?

1. Fibrous attachment from granuloma to optic nerve with dragged vessels.

2. The differential diagnosis for temporally dragged disc is toxocariasis, FEVR, and congenital falciform fold. Other causes of retinal dragging include ROP, incontinential pigmenti, and X-linked retinoschisis, and may also occur in adults with traction retinal detachment, proliferative vitreoretinopathy, and epiretinal membrane.

3. Toxocariasis (ocular larva migrans).

4. Ocular larva migrans has three clinical presentations depending on patient age at time of infection:

   Chronic endophthalmitis: 2–9 years of age; granulomatous posterior uveitis with vitreous exudate and cyclitic membrane, which often leads to destruction of the globe.

   Localized granuloma: 6–14 years of age; granuloma in macula or peripapillary area, no inflammation, strabismus, nonprogressive.

   Peripheral granuloma: 6–40 year of age; granuloma in periphery with fibrotic strand often to disc, strabismus, nonprogressive.

   Visceral larva migrans does not have eye involvement.

5. Infection due to the second-stage larval form of the common roundworm *toxocara canis* or *toxocara cati*. The nematode lives in dog or cat intestines. The mature adult releases eggs that are passed in the stool. Contact with infected fecal material leads to human infection (more common in children and young adults), but the roundworm cannot sexually mature. Local inflammatory reactions lead to encapsulation of the worm. Seroprevalence has been estimated at 14% in the US with higher prevalence in the South. Risk factors include contact with puppies and kittens and eating dirt (pica); older dogs are less likely to cause infection.

6. Antiparasitic therapy with albendazole or thiabendazole is unproven. Treatment is largely based on reducing the inflammation using steroids. In the presence of inflammation, dilating drops should also be used. In 25% of cases, vitreoretinal surgery to treat ERM, traction RD, and/or vitreous hemorrhage is required.

A 10-year-old girl is examined for a new pair of glasses and is noted to have a left head turn.

1. What abnormality does this child have?

2. What additional history and testing would you obtain?

Additional information: the mother reports a normal pregnancy and full-term delivery, and says that her daughter is healthy and takes no medication but that her left eye looks smaller than the right. There is no family history of eye disease, and the only past ocular history is low myopia for which she wears glasses at school. On exam, the BSCVA is 20/20 OU, the eyes appear straight in primary position, extraocular motility is full OD and limited in both abduction and adduction OS as demonstrated in the photos. There is a small left head turn to improve fusion.

3. What is the diagnosis?

4. How is this condition classified?

5. What is the etiology?

6. What other findings occur?

7. What is the treatment?

1. The photos demonstrate limited abduction and adduction OS. There is also narrowing of the left palpebral fissure and elevation of the left eye with attempted adduction, and widening of the left palpebral fissure on attempted abduction.

2. A complete history must be obtained including birth history (ie, prematurity), past ocular history (visual acuity, glasses use, any trauma, surgery, strabismus, patching/penalization), family history of eye disorders, past medical history and medications. A complete eye exam should be performed with attention to visual acuity, refraction, fusion and motility tests (cover-uncover, and alternate cover).

3. Duane's retraction syndrome type 3.

4. There are three types (1>3>2), the left eye is affected more commonly, and 20% are bilateral:

   Type 1: limited abduction, esotropia in primary position

   Type 2: limited adduction, exotropia in primary position

   Type 3: limited abduction and adduction.

5. Congenital agenesis or hypoplasia of the abducens nerve (CN 6) and abnormal innervation of the lateral rectus muscle by a branch of CN 3.

6. In addition to limitations of horizontal motility, cocontraction of the medial and lateral rectus muscles result in globe retraction and narrowing of the palpebral fissure. The palpebral fissure of the affected side narrows on adduction and widens on abduction. Vertical deviations referred to as upshoots and downshoots (leash phenomenon) often occur, and the patient may have a head turn to fuse. Other associated abnormalities are deafness, crocodile tears, syndromes (Goldenhar's syndrome, Klippel–Feil syndrome, Wildervanck's syndrome, fetal alcohol syndrome, cat-eye syndrome), and other findings of prenatal thalidomide exposure.

7. Any refractive error should be corrected and amblyopia should be treated. Otherwise, Duane's syndrome usually does not require treatment, but indications for muscle surgery include a deviation in primary position, abnormal head position, or significant upshoot or downshoot.

A 6-year-old boy presents with unilateral leukocoria.

1. What findings are evident in the photo?
2. What is the differential diagnosis?

Additonal information: the FA shows:

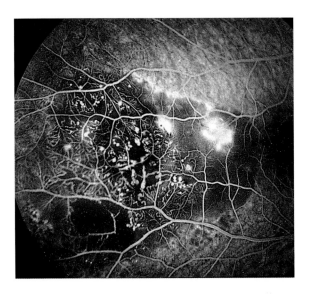

3. Describe the FA findings. What is the diagnosis?
4. What is the staging of this disease?
5. How would you treat this patient?
6. What is the prognosis?

1. Retinal telangiectasia with extensive leaking telangiectatic vessels, massive lipid exudates, and an exudative retinal detachment.

2. Coats disease, PHPV, retinoblastoma, angiomatosis retinae.

3. The FA demonstrates large telangiectatic vessels and numerous leaking aneurysms ("light bulb" dilatations). This is the classic presentation of Coats disease.

4. There are two staging schema for Coats disease:

   Gomez–Morales Staging
   Stage I: Focal exudates
   Stage II: Massive exudation
   Stage III: Partial exudative retinal detachment
   Stage IV: Total retinal detachment
   Stage V: Complications

   Sigelman Staging
   Stage I: Only telangiactasia
   Stage II: Focal exudates
   Stage III: Partial exudative retinal detachment
   Stage IV: Total retinal detachment
   Stage V: Complications

   Coats disease represents the severe form of a spectrum of disease. The milder form is Leber's miliary aneurysms, which occurs in older individuals, affects men and women equally, and is usually bilateral.

4. Laser treatment, cryotherapy, and anti-VEGF injections have all been tried.

5. The prognosis depends on the stage of the disease. The older the patient at presentation the better the prognosis; often the prognosis is poor when presenting before age 3 years old.

A 5-day-old infant is found to have redness and discharge from both eyes.

1. What questions would you ask the mother?
2. What is the diagnosis?
3. What are the possible etiologies?

Additional information: the mother reports a normal full-term vaginal delivery and no premature rupture of the membranes. She has no history of HSV or GC. The infant received topical erythromycin ointment OU at the hospital and has not had any medication since and has no other signs or symptoms of infection. The redness and discharge began 1 day ago, and the discharge is yellow and moderate in quantity.

4. What is the most likely cause?
5. How would you work up this infant?
6. What is the appropriate treatment?

1. It is helpful to know when the redness and discharge began. What is the quantity and quality of the discharge? Does the baby have a fever or any other signs of infection (runny nose, cough, rash, lethargy, emesis, etc.)? Has the baby received any medications? Was the birth vaginal or C-section? Were there any complications? Does the mother have any communicable diseases?

2. Conjunctivitis, specifically ophthalmia neonatorum.

3. Chemical (silver nitrate 1% solution), bacterial, viral (HSV), and chlamydial (neonatal inclusion conjunctivitis).

4. Bacterial, most likely *H. influenzae*, *S. pneumoniae*, or *M. catarrhalis*.

5. Gram stain and culture to determine the organism.

6. Empiric topical antibiotic (bacitracin, erythromycin, or gentamicin ointment) for 7 days; may require systemic antibiotic for extraocular involvement (ie, otitis media).

A 26-year-old man has a history of reduced vision.

1. What is the differential diagnosis?
2. What diagnostic tests should you perform?

Additional information: the OCT shows:

3. What is the diagnosis?
4. What is the etiology?
5. Describe the pathophysiology and stages of this disease.

1. Best disease or vitelliform macular dystrophy (most likely), adult foveomacular vitelliform dystrophy, age-related macular degeneration, North Carolina macular dystrophy, macular coloboma, dominant drusen, central serous chorioretinopathy, solar retinopathy, macular hole, toxoplasmosis, myopic degeneration, old foveal hemorrhage, syphilis, autosomal recessive bestrophinopathy, autosomal dominant vitreoretinochoroidopathy.

2. Usually diagnosed by clinical examination but EOG shows an abnormal Arden ratio with normal ERG. OCT nicely demonstrates the vitelliform lesion. FA shows hypofluoresent blockage of the vitelliform lesion. Fundus autofluorescence shows hyperautofluorescence in the early stages and hypoautofluorescence during the atrophic stage. Genetic testing for the *BEST1* gene on the long arm of chromosome 11, which encodes the transmembrane protein bestrophin1.

3. The OCT is consistent with Best disease.

4. Best disease is a hereditary (autosomal dominant) macular dystrophy caused by mutations in the *BEST1* gene on chromosome 11q12-q13.1.

5. Primary disturbance of the RPE leading to a build up of lipofuscin within the RPE and subRPE space. In late stage, secondary loss of overlying photoreceptors occurs. There are five stages of Best disease:

   Stage I (Previtelliform): normal or only subtle RPE changes (tiny, central honeycomb structure centrally). Normal vision with abnormal EOG.

   Stage II (Vitelliform): well circumscribed, round, classic "egg-yolk" appearance in the fovea. 30% have ectopic lesions. Normal vision or mild vision loss (20/20–20/50).

   Stage III (Pseudohypopyon): layering of lipufuscin as material breaks through RPE into subretinal space. Vision similar to stage II.

   Stage IV (Vitelleruptive): breakup of lipofuscin material leads to "scrambled egg" stage. Vision is mildly decreased from earlier stages (20/20–20/100).

   Stage V (Atrophic): Central retinal atrophy with disappearance of lipofuscin material. Vision worse (20/80–20/200).

   Stage VI (CNV): Choroidal neovascularization occurs in approximately 20% of patients.

A 65-year-old man notices a red bump on his right upper eyelid that has been enlarging for the past 6 weeks. He initially applied warm compresses once a day without any improvement.

1. What do you think this represents, and what is the differential diagnosis?
2. What would be your next step?

Additional information: the pathology shows:

3. What is the diagnosis?
4. How would you treat this patient?
5. How would the treatment differ for sebaceous gland carcinoma?

1. The lesion appears to be a squamous cell carcinoma or keratoacanthoma, but other possibilities are basal cell carcinoma, sebaceous gland carcinoma, inflamed actinic keratosis, tricholemmoma, and Merkel cell tumor.

2. Biopsy.

3. Keratoacanthoma, which is classified as a squamous cell carcinoma.

4. Complete excision of the lesion.

5. Sebaceous gland carcinoma requires wide excision with frozen section and conjunctival map biopsy. Exenteration is performed for orbital extension or pagetoid spread. Radiotherapy is used for palliation.

A 26-year-old man complains of a red, painful left eye. He is sensitive to bright light but does not have any change in vision.

1. What is the differential diagnosis?
2. What additional questions would you ask this patient?

Additional information: the patient reports no previous ocular history and does not have any medical problems. Review of systems is negative, and he denies any history of foreign travel or sexually transmitted disease. Exam shows a tender, red, immobile scleral nodule, mild anterior chamber cell and flare, and normal IOP and fundus.

3. What is the diagnosis?
4. What are the different types of scleritis?
5. What are the possible etiologies?
6. What pharmacologic test can differentiate between scleritis and episcleritis?
7. What disease causes anterior necrotizing scleritis without inflammation (scleromalacia perforans)?
8. What are the signs of posterior scleritis?
9. How would you manage this patient?

1. Episcleritis, scleritis, Tenon's cyst, lymphoid lesion, and myositis.

2. Has he had any previous episodes? Does he have any systemic diseases (specifically collagen vascular or autoimmune)? Has he had any eye trauma or surgery? Any recent sinus problems, difficulty in breathing, joint pain, fever or night sweats? Any foreign travel? Does he have a history of a sexually transmitted disease?

3. Nodular anterior scleritis.

4. Anterior (98%) and posterior (2%). Anterior can be diffuse, nodular, or necrotizing with or without inflammation.

5. There is a systemic association in 50% of cases and 30% of cases have a collagen vascular disease (rheumatoid arthritis, ankylosing spondylitis, systemic lupus erythematosus, polyarteritis nodosa, Wegener's granulomatosis, or relapsing polychondritis). Other etiologies are herpes zoster, syphilis, tuberculosis, leprosy, gout, porphyria, and idiopathic.

6. Topical phenylephrine 2.5% will blanch the injected area if it is due to episcleritis but will not if it is due to scleritis.

7. Rheumatoid arthritis.

8. Chorioretinal folds, serous retinal detachments, vitritis, optic disc edema, and "T-sign" and thickened sclera on B-scan ultrasound.

9. This patient requires a systemic workup including: CBC with differential, ESR, RF, ANA, ANCA (antineutrophil cytoplasmic antibody), VDRL or RPR (rapid plasma reagin), FTA-ABS or MHA-TP (microhemagglutination assay for *Treponema pallidum*), uric acid, BUN (blood urea nitrogen), PPD (purified protein derivative of tuberculin), and chest X-ray. Treatment is with oral NSAIDs. Systemic steroids, antibiotics, and possibly immunosuppressive agents may be necessary depending on the underlying etiology.

A 55-year-old woman complains of a bump on her eye.

1. What is the differential diagnosis?
2. What would be the next step?

Additional information: the pathology shows:

3. What is the diagnosis and why?
4. How would you treat this patient if the pathology had shown squamous cell carcinoma?

1. This conjunctival lesion could be a pinguecula, papilloma, conjunctival intraepithelial neoplasia, squamous cell carcinoma, or a lymphoid tumor.

2. Excisional biopsy.

3. CIN (conjunctival intraepithelial neoplasia), because the atypical cells are confined to the epithelium without penetration of the basement membrane.

4. Wide surgical excision with episclerectomy, corneal epitheliectomy with 100% alcohol, and cryotherapy to the bed of the lesion. Consider topical 5-fluorouracil, topical mitomycin C, or interferon alpha-2b (topical or subconjunctival). Intraocular involvement requires enucleation, and orbital involvement requires exenteration with radiation.

A 62-year-old woman reports that her right eye has been irritated, red, and tearing for months. Artificial tears help briefly but do not really alleviate the scratchy sensation she experiences.

1. What are the diagnosis and possible etiologies?
2. What other history would be helpful?
3. What would you look for on exam to help determine the cause?
4. How would you manage this patient?

1. Entropion. The etiologies include cicatricial, involutional, and spastic.

2. Any previous ocular or periocular trauma, surgery, or disorder?

3. Lid tone (snapback test), lower lid margin position (sagging), and ability to rotate the lower lid by pressing on the inferior tarsal border.

4. The ocular surface must be protected from the inturned lashes with frequent instillation of lubricating drops, gels, and/or ointments. Surgical repair is often necessary and the most appropriate procedure depends on the type of entropion:

   Cicatricial: excision of scar with possible anterior lamellar resection or recession, tarsal fracture, tarsal graft, or conjunctival/mucous membrane grafts. Consider removing lashes.

   Involutional: lid taping, thermal cautery, or Quickert suture; horizontal or vertical lid shortening; and/or lid retractor repair.

   Spastic: lid taping, thermal cautery, Botox injection, Quickert suture, lateral tightening with transconjunctival advancement of lid retractors.

A 38-year-old man complains of intermittent red, irritated eyes for several years. His symptoms are worse in the morning. His past medical history is positive for high cholesterol and moderate obesity.

1. What abnormality is shown?
2. What additional history would be helpful?

Additional information: the patient has no past ocular history, never wore contact lenses, and has no allergies. He denies any difficulty with his vision, can only describe his eye discomfort as "irritating," and sometimes has a little discharge in his eyes when he wakes up. Artificial tears help but only briefly. Exam reveals mild conjunctival injection and a papillary reaction of the superior tarsal conjunctiva. There is no lid margin disease, discharge, or corneal staining. The tear meniscus, tear break-up time, and Schirmer's test are normal.

3. What specific finding would you look for on exam?
4. This finding is present, what is the diagnosis?
5. What other conditions are associated with this syndrome?
6. What is the treatment?

1. Superior tarsal conjunctival papillae.

2. Is there any discharge? What is the primary symptom (itching, burning, or foreign body sensation)? Is there any change in vision? Does he wear contact lenses? Does he have any allergies? Has he used any treatment?

3. Easily everted upper eyelids.

4. Floppy eyelid syndrome.

5. Obesity, sleep apnea, keratoconus, and eyelid rubbing.

6. Tape, patch, or shield the lids for sleeping. Consider surgery with a horizontal lid-tightening procedure.

A 24-year-old woman reports red, itchy eyes for the past month. Her primary physician treated her with gentamicin eye drops for 2 weeks with no improvement. She was then given blephamide for 1 week, which helped, but her symptoms recurred when she stopped the drops. She has not used any eye drops for 1 week. She denies any change in vision or mucus discharge.

1. What is the diagnosis?
2. What are the possible etiologies?
3. What are the etiologies of membranous conjunctivitis?
4. What other questions would you ask this patient?
5. What other findings would you look for on exam?

Additional information: she recently had a flareup of sinusitis but has not had a cold or been around known contacts with an eye infection. She does not wear contact lenses and does not have any known allergies. She denies having a STD. There are no eyelid lesions, subepithelial corneal infiltrates, or preauricular lymphadenopathy.

6. How would you work up this patient?

Additional information: the conjunctival scraping shows:

7. What is the diagnosis?
8. What is the treatment?

1. Follicular conjunctivitis.

2. Virus (adenovirus, HSV), chlamydia, molluscum, and drug reaction.

3. A true membrane is caused by *Streptococcus, Gonococcus, Corynebacterium diphtheriae,* Stevens–Johnson syndrome, and chemical burns.

4. Has she had a recent upper respiratory infection or fever? Has she been around anyone with an eye infection? Does she wear contact lenses? Has she ever had a sexually transmitted disease?

5. Preauricular lymphadenopathy, eyelid lesions, pseudomembrane on the inferior tarsal conjunctiva, subconjunctival hemorrhage, subepithelial infiltrates in the cornea.

6. Obtain a conjunctival culture and scraping.

7. Chlamydial conjunctivitis. The scraping shows basophilic cytoplasmic inclusion bodies in epithelial cells.

8. Systemic and topical antibiotics with tetracyclines or erythromycins (azithromycin), and also treat all sexual partners.

An 18-year-old man complains of a red and painful right eye with blurry vision. It has gotten worse over the past 4 days since he was gardening and thinks he got scratched by a plant branch.

1. What is the most likely diagnosis?

2. How would you manage this patient?

3. What are the indications for a corneal biopsy?

Additional information: KOH prep is positive and a Gram's stain of scraping from the ulcer shows the following organism:

4. What is the diagnosis?

5. What are the characteristic findings of this type of keratitis?

6. What is the treatment?

1. Microbial keratitis, probably fungal or bacterial.

2. Perform corneal cultures and smears of the ulcer and start empiric antibiotic treatment with topical fortified antibiotics (cefazolin and tobramycin) alternating every hour initially, and a cycloplegic drop. Ask the patient about contact lens wear and if he does wear contacts the lens and case should be cultured as well. This vision-threatening corneal infection initially requires daily follow-up monitoring the vision, IOP, size, depth, and density of the corneal infiltrate, and presence and size of any overlying epithelial defect. Therapy should be adjusted based on the culture and sensitivity results. Confocal microscopy if available is useful for identifying fungi and *Acanthamoeba*.

3. A biopsy should be considered for progressive disease, a culture-negative ulcer, or a deep abscess.

4. Fungal keratitis. The scraping shows branching fungal hyphae of *Fusarium*.

5. Fungal ulcers usually have feathery edges, endothelial plaque, satellite infiltrates, and may penetrate Descemet's membrane.

6. Topical antifungal (natamycin, amphotericin B, miconazole, or voriconazole) and cycloplegic drops. Topical steroids are contraindicated. For severe infection, add systemic antifungal (ketoconazole or amphotericin B).

A 46-year-old man has a history of multiple ocular surgeries for glaucoma and cataract. He reports deterioration of his vision in the left eye. He notices a white film on the eye but denies any pain.

1. What is the diagnosis?
2. What is the pathology?
3. With which ocular disease is this most commonly associated?
4. How would you treat this patient?
5. What is the prognosis?

1. Is there a family history of eye disease or surgery (ie, corneal transplant)? Does the vision fluctuate throughout the day or with different geographic locations (worse in the morning or in humid environments)?

2. Corneal pachymetry and specular microscopy.

3. Fuchs' endothelial dystrophy.

4. Medical treatment consists of hypertonic ointment at bedtime and drops during the day. A course of topical steroids may be helpful. Surgical treatment is corneal transplantation (EK [endothelial keratoplasty; DSAEK, DMEK] or PK [penetrating keratoplasty]).

5. In addition to graft rejection, failure, hemorrhage, infection, and glaucoma, other specific complications are graft dislocation for EK and nonhealing epithelial defect, wound dehiscence, and irregular astigmatism for PK.

A 42-year-old man has a history of poor vision. The appearance of his right eye is shown.

1. What is the most likely diagnosis?

2. What are the etiologies?

3. What other findings are seen in congenital syphilis?

4. What triad of findings characterizes Cogan's syndrome?

5. What is the treatment of active disease?

6. What ocular treatment would you offer this patient?

1. Interstitial keratitis (IK).

2. IK is usually infectious. The most common infections are syphilis, HSV (herpes simplex virus), and tuberculosis; also VZV (varicella zoster virus), mumps, rubella, leprosy, and onchocerciasis. Other causes include sarcoidosis and Cogan's syndrome.

3. Optic nerve atrophy, salt-and-pepper fundus, deafness, notched teeth, saddle nose, and sabre shins.

4. IK, vertigo, and hearing loss.

5. Topical steroid and cycloplegic drops for the corneal inflammation, and treat the underlying condition.

6. Chronic, inactive interstitial keratitis with corneal scarring can be treated with a lamellar or penetrating keratoplasty.

A 26-year-old woman complains of red, irritated eyes for 3 weeks. She wears disposable contact lenses but cannot tolerate them for more than an hour or two. Yesterday she noticed some mucous discharge in the morning. Her primary doctor gave her an antibiotic ointment, which she puts in her eyes twice a day, and she also uses artificial tears once or twice a day. Exam shows scant white mucus strands in the inferior fornix OD and minimal conjunctival injection OU.

1. What is the differential diagnosis?

Additional information: the eyelids and tear film are normal. There are no conjunctival follicles on the bulbar or inferior palpebral surface, and there is no corneal staining or infiltrate.

2. What other finding would you look for on exam to make the diagnosis?

1. Blepharoconjunctivitis, acute bacterial conjunctivitis, conjunctivitis due to allergy or toxicity to the antibiotic ointment, giant papillary conjunctivitis (GPC), contact lens overwear, or corneal ulcer.

2. Giant papillae on the superior tarsal conjunctiva by everting the upper eyelids.

Additional information: this maneuver reveals the following:

3. What is the diagnosis?

4. How would you treat her?

5. Besides contact lenses, what are other causes of this disorder?

3. GPC.

4. Treatment is to discontinue contact lens wear, use a combination mast cell stabilizer/antihistamine drop, and, depending on the severity, also add a topical steroid. If a steroid is used, the IOP must be monitored.

5. GPC is mainly associated with contact lens wear, but other causes include a foreign body, exposed suture, or prosthesis.

An asymptomatic 57-year-old woman presents for a routine eye exam. Her left eye is shown in the photo.

1. What is the diagnosis, and what term is used to refer to this type of lesion?

2. What other ocular findings would you specifically look for on exam?

3. How would you work up this patient?

4. What is the treatment?

5. What is the risk of systemic lymphoma in patients with an ocular lymphoid lesion?

1. This is a conjunctival lymphoid tumor and is commonly referred to as a salmon patch.

2. Visual changes, limited ocular motility, proptosis, and lacrimal gland swelling to evaluate for orbital involvement, and lid examination to evaluate for eyelid involvement.

3. The patient requires a medical/oncology consultation and workup to determine whether there is orbital or systemic involvement. Tests include CBC with differential, serum protein electrophoresis (SPEP), ESR, CT scan (orbital, thoracic, and abdominal), and bone scan.

4. The next step is a biopsy and evaluation of the fresh specimen with immunohistochemical studies to determine the type of lymphoid tumor (benign reactive lymphoid hyperplasia, atypical lymphoid hyperplasia, or lymphoma [50% are mucosa-associated lymphoid tissue (MALT)]), since they cannot be distinguished clinically. Treatment is based on the diagnosis and extent of involvement, and is with external beam radiation, chemotherapy, and surgery.

5. The risk is 67% for an eyelid lesion, 35% for an orbit lesion, and 20% for a conjunctiva lesion.

A 48-year-old man reports a tender swollen left upper eyelid and tearing for 8 days. He denies any trauma or change in vision.

1. What is the differential diagnosis?
2. What other questions would you ask him?

Additional information: he does have a fever and reports some discharge from the eye, but there is no diplopia. On exam, he has palpable preauricular lymphadenopathy. His vision is 20/25 in both eyes, pupillary response, extraocular motility, and confrontation visual fields are normal. External exam shows a firm, tender mass of the lateral upper eyelid. Anterior and posterior segment exams are normal. An orbital CT scan shows:

3. What is the diagnosis?
4. What are the possible etiologies?
5. How would you work up this patient?
6. What is the treatment?
7. If this lacrimal gland mass were a neoplasm, what would be the differential diagnosis?
8. What is the treatment of a benign mixed tumor?

1. Preseptal or orbital cellulitis, chalazion, eyelid tumor, dacryoadenitis, or lacrimal gland tumor.

2. Has he had a recent infection or fever, or trauma to the lid? Does he have double vision? Is there any discharge?

3. Acute dacryoadenitis.

4. Infection due to *Staphylococcus*, mumps, EBV (Epstein–Barr virus), VZV, *Neisseria gonorrhoeae*.

5. Obtain a culture and Gram stain of the discharge, CBC with differential, and possibly blood cultures.

6. Treat the underlying infection with the appropriate systemic antimicrobial agents. He may require incision and drainage or excision.

7. Lacrimal gland tumors are lymphoproliferative (50%) or epithelial (50%). Half of the epithelial tumors are pleomorphic adenomas (benign mixed tumors) and half are malignant (adenoid cystic carcinomas and malignant mixed tumors).

8. Complete en bloc excision without biopsy because rupture of the pseudocapsule can result in recurrence and malignant transformation.

A 78-year-old woman says she scratched her eyelid 3 weeks ago and it bled, but it hasn't healed yet.

1. What do you suspect this lesion represents?
2. What is the differential diagnosis?

Additional information: a biopsy reveals the following pathology.

3. What is the diagnosis?
4. What are the characteristic findings of this tumor?
5. What are the characteristic findings of sebaceous gland carcinoma?
6. What is the treatment for BCC?
7. Which location on the eyelids has the worst prognosis?

1. This is suspicious for a skin cancer, most likely basal cell carcinoma (BCC).

2. Other malignant epithelial tumors of the eyelid are squamous cell carcinoma, keratoacanthoma, and malignant melanoma.

3. Basal cell carcinoma.

4. The more common nodular BCC has raised, pearly, nodular borders, and telangiectasia. There may be central ulceration (rodent ulcer) and distortion of the surrounding normal eyelid architecture with scarring and eyelash loss. The morpheaform BCC, which is rarer but more aggressive, appears as a firm, flat plaque with ulceration and indistinct borders that penetrates in to the dermis and can have pagetoid spread.

5. Sebaceous gland carcinoma is highly malignant and appears as a hard, yellow nodule. It can masquerade as chronic unilateral blepharitis or recurrent chalazion with thickened, red lid margin inflammation and loss of lashes.

6. Wide surgical excision with frozen section margin control, Mohs' micrographic surgery, and may require cryotherapy or radiation therapy. Canthal tumors require orbital CT scan to assess posterior involvement. Exenteration is performed for orbital extension.

7. Medial canthus because the tumor often extends deeper and can involve the lacrimal drainage system.

A 71-year-old woman complains of dry eyes for years. The appearance of her ocular surface is seen in the photo.

1. What are the findings and possible etiologies?

2. How do acid and alkali burns differ?

3. What is the acute treatment for chemical burns?

4. How are chemical burns graded?

5. What are the complications of chemical burns?

6. What are the most common causes of Stevens–Johnson syndrome?

7. What other questions would you like to ask this patient?

Additional information: she has hypertension, which is controlled on medication. She has never been hospitalized and denies any drug allergies or reactions. Review of systems does reveal dysphagia. Past ocular history is negative except for cataract surgery OS 10 years ago. Since then, her dry eye has gotten worse.

8. What is the diagnosis?

9. What would a conjunctival biopsy show?

10. What is the treatment?

11. What is the prognosis?

1. Symblepharon, which can be caused by chemical burn, Stevens–Johnson syndrome (SJS), ocular cicatricial pemphigoid, trachoma, herpes zoster, atopic keratoconjunctivitis, scleroderma, graft versus host disease.

2. Acid tends to cause less severe injury than alkali. Acid denatures and precipitates proteins, which form a barrier to further penetration. Alkali denatures but does not precipitate proteins, and also saponifies fats (disrupts lipid membranes), causing deeper penetration into ocular tissues.

3. Copious irrigation checking pH level, débridement (any necrotic conjunctiva and particulate matter), frequent lubrication, topical antibiotic and cycloplegic, consider topical (10%) and oral sodium ascorbate (aids collagen synthesis and scavenges superoxide radicals), collagenase inhibitor (acetylcysteine or EDTA), steroids (for first 5–10 days only to reduce corneal and intraocular inflammation and help prevent symblepharon, but can enhance collagenase-induced corneal melting, which often begins 1–2 weeks after injury), may require control of elevated IOP, bandage contact lens, or tarsorrhaphy. Symblepharon lysis is performed with a glass rod.

4. Mild to severe based on degree of corneal damage and ischemia:

   Grade I: corneal epithelial damage, no ischemia

   Grade II: stromal haze but iris details visible, ischemia < 1/3 of limbus

   Grade III: total corneal epithelial loss, stromal haze, iris obscured

   Grade IV: opaque cornea, ischemia >1/2 of limbus

5. Dry eye, symblepharon, entropion, anterior segment ischemia, cataract, glaucoma, uveitis, neurotrophic keratitis, corneal ulceration, scarring, and perforation.

6. SJS is usually drug-induced (sulfonamides, penicillin, aspirin, barbiturates, isoniazid, phenytoin) or infectious (HSV, *Mycoplasma*, adenovirus, *Streptococcus*).

7. What is the past medical and ocular history? Is there any previous eye surgery, injury, or infection? Any severe reactions to medications? Does she have any unusual skin lesions or difficulty swallowing or breathing?

8. Ocular cicatricial pemphigoid (OCP).

9. Immunoglobulin and complement deposition in the basement membrane.

10. Treatment is with lubrication and systemic steroids or immunosuppressive therapy (ie, dapsone, cyclophosphamide). Patients may require surgery for entropion, trichiasis, symblepharon, ankyloblepharon, and corneal scarring.

11. OCP is a chronic, progressive disease. Surgery can cause exacerbations and should be used with caution. PK has a poor success rate, and keratoprosthesis also has limited success, but is used in end-stage disease.

A 56-year-old woman complains of a red painful right eye and blurry vision for several weeks. On exam, there is moderate ciliary injection, peripheral thinning of the cornea, and a mild anterior chamber reaction.

1. What is the differential diagnosis of peripheral corneal thinning?
2. What findings help distinguish Mooren's ulcer from Terrien's marginal degeneration?
3. What additional history would you like from this patient?

Additional information: further history is unremarkable. The patient does not have blepharitis.

4. How would you work up this patient?
5. The C-ANCA is positive. What is the diagnosis and treatment?

1. Mooren's ulcer, marginal keratolysis, staphylococcal marginal keratitis, Terrien's marginal degeneration.

2. Mooren's ulcer is painful and has an undermined leading edge with an overhanging margin, absent epithelium in active areas, and may have conjunctival injection.

   Terrien's marginal degeneration is bilateral, painless, and has a leading edge of lipid, steep central edge, sloping peripheral edge, intact epithelium, and superficial vascularization.

3. Does she have any past ocular or medical history? Has she had any previous similar episodes? If she does not have any medical problems, then a careful review of systems should be obtained with attention to autoimmune and collagen vascular disease symptoms.

4. Mooren's ulcer is a diagnosis of exclusion whereas marginal keratolysis is due to systemic disease, so it is necessary to order the following lab tests: CBC with differential, ESR, RF, ANA, ANCA, BUN, creatinine, and urinalysis. If infection is suspected, then culture and smears should be obtained.

5. Wegener's granulomatosis, which requires systemic steroids and immunosuppressive therapy (cyclophosphamide). The eye should be treated with lubrication, punctal occlusion, and possibly tarsorrhaphy to heal the epithelium and prevent further corneal melting. Topical cyclosporine, acetylcysteine, and conjunctival recession or resection may be helpful. Tectonic or penetrating keratoplasty may be required for significant thinning.

A 44-year-old Caucasian man who has not had an eye exam in 10 years says that he is having more difficulty reading. His eye exam is normal except for the lesion shown above.

1. What are the most likely diagnoses?

2. What are the characteristics of each?

3. What other history would be relevant?

Additional information: he has not noticed it before and has no history or family history of skin cancer.

4. What is the indication for biopsy of PAM?

5. A biopsy confirms the diagnosis of PAM with atypia. What is the treatment and prognosis?

1. This pigmented lesion is probably a conjunctival nevus or primary acquired melanosis (PAM); malignant melanoma is less likely.

2. Nevus: a discrete, elevated, variably pigmented lesion that contains cysts. It may enlarge during puberty and is rarely malignant.

   PAM: a patchy, diffuse, flat lesion with indistinct margins that does not contain cysts. It may grow (nodular thickening) and involve the cornea.

   Malignant melanoma: a nodular, variably pigmented lesion with blood vessels that does not contain cysts. It may arise from PAM (70%), a preexisting nevus (20%), or de novo (10%).

3. Has he noticed the pigmentation and if so, for how long? Has it changed in color or size? Does he have a history of skin cancer, specifically melanoma?

4. Nodular thickening is the indication for excisional biopsy.

5. PAM with nodular thickening is treated with excisional biopsy and cryotherapy. Recurrence can be treated with topical interferon alpha-2b or mitomycin C. Complete excision is required for malignancy. PAM has a low risk for progression to melanoma: PAM without or with mild atypia has no risk, and PAM with severe atypia has a 13% risk of malignant transformation. The greatest risk is the extent of the lesion in clock hours.

62.0	Power: 57.4D
59.5	(5.88 mm)
57.0	From vertex:
54.5	Dist 0.00 mm
52.0	S-merid 0°
49.5	
47.0	SimK Values:
44.5	58.75D @112
42.0	48.75D @22
39.5	
37.0	OD
34.5	
Diopter	11/20/08 11:11 AM

Axial Map

Power: 42.8D	47.0
(7.88 mm)	46.0
From vertex:	45.0
Dist 0.00 mm	44.0
S-merid 0°	43.0
	42.0
SimK Values:	41.0
43.37D @94	40.0
42.12D @4	39.0
	38.0
OS	37.0
	36.0
11/20/08 11:11 AM	Diopter

Axial Map

A 28-year-old man with myopia and astigmatism is interested in LASIK. He does not wear contact lenses. His corneal topography is shown.

1. What is the diagnosis?

2. What is the pathology?

3. Are there any associations?

4. What signs would you look for on exam?

5. How is this condition diagnosed with corneal topography (CVK)?

6. What other conditions may have a similar appearance on CVK?

7. What are the treatment options?

8. How is hydrops treated?

1. Keratoconus (KC).

2. KC is a bilateral, asymmetric, noninflammatory, cone-shaped deformity of the cornea due to progressive central or paracentral stromal thinning with breaks in Bowman's membrane and superficial scarring. Hydrops is acute corneal edema due to a break in Descemet's membrane.

3. KC is typically associated with eye rubbing, Down syndrome, and connective tissue disease. Ocular associations include retinitis pigmentosa, atopic keratoconjunctivitis (AKC), VKC, Leber's congenital amaurosis, floppy eyelid syndrome, congenital hereditary endothelial dystrophy (CHED), and posterior polymorphous dystrophy (PPMD).

4. Irregular astigmatism (decreased visual acuity, scissors reflex on retinoscopy, steep keratometry with irregular mires, abnormal corneal topography), apical corneal thinning and scarring, Fleischer ring (epithelial iron deposition around base of cone), Vogt's striae (deep, stromal, vertical stress lines at apex of cone), prominent corneal nerves, Munson's sign (protrusion of lower lid with downgaze), and Rizzuti's sign (triangle of light on iris from penlight beam focused by cone), may have hydrops (opaque edematous cornea, ciliary injection, and anterior chamber cells and flare).

5. Characteristic pattern of irregular astigmatism: central or inferior steepening in KC, and similar pattern or asymmetric skewed bow-tie pattern in form fruste or KC suspects. Most CVK devices contain KC analysis software.

   Three specific parameters can be used to aid in the diagnosis:

   1. Central corneal power >47.2 D.

   2. Difference in corneal power between fellow eyes >0.92 D.

   3. I-S value (difference between average inferior and superior corneal powers 3 mm from the center of the cornea): >1.4 D.

6. Contact-lens-induced corneal warpage, keratectasia (after laser vision correction), and pellucid marginal degeneration.

7. Depending on the severity, glasses or rigid gas permeable contact lenses, corneal collagen cross linking, intracorneal ring segments (Intacs), and penetrating keratoplasty. LASIK is contraindicated.

8. Treatment for hydrops is supportive with topical steroids, cycloplegic, and bandage contact lens.

A 36-year-old woman comes in for a routine exam. The appearance of her corneas is shown.

1. What is the diagnosis?

2. What is the pattern of inheritance?

3. What other anterior corneal dystrophies may have a similar appearance with tiny dots or subepithelial scarring?

4. What is the pathology of each?

5. What are the possible sequelae of this patient's disorder?

6. What is the treatment?

1. Epithelial basement membrane dystrophy (EBMD; anterior basement membrane dystrophy [ABMD], map-dot-fingerprint [MDF] dystrophy), the most common anterior corneal dystrophy.

2. Autosomal dominant in isolated familial cases, but the majority is degenerative.

3. Meesmann dystrophy, Reis–Bucklers dystrophy, and Thiel–Behnke dystrophy.

4. Epithelial basement membrane dystrophy: abnormal epithelial adhesion causes intraepithelial and subepithelial basement membrane reduplication with intraepithelial microcysts (dots) and subepithelial ridges and lines (map-like and fingerprint-like).

    Meesmann dystrophy: epithelial cells contain PAS-positive material (peculiar substance) and the epithelial basement membrane is thickened.

    Reis–Bucklers dystrophy: absence of Bowman's layer, replacement by granular irregular deposits extending in to stroma.

    Thiel–Behnke dystrophy: replacement of Bowman's layer by fibrocellular material in a pathognomonic wavy "sawtooth" pattern; curly fibers on electron microscopy

5. Recurrent erosions (10%) or decreased vision (from subepithelial scarring).

6. Asymptomatic patients require no treatment.

    Erosions are treated with lubrication and hypertonic saline (Muro 128 5% ointment at bedtime for up to 1 year) after the epithelial defect heals. For recurrences, consider a bandage contact lens, epithelial débridement, anterior stromal puncture, or PTK. Also, consider treatment with matrix metalloproteinase-9 inhibitors (oral doxycycline and topical steroids).

    Subepithelial scarring causing decreased vision or monocular diplopia is treated with débridement.

A 32-year-old woman reports a painful eye for 2 weeks and blurry vision. Past ocular history is notable for myopia and contact lens wear. She has never had a problem with contact lenses before and stopped wearing the lenses when the irritation started. Her past medical and ocular histories are negative. She has been using Viroptic for the last 12 days but her vision has gotten worse and she is very sensitive to light. Examination shows minimal conjunctival injection, paracentral anterior corneal haze, and punctate corneal staining.

1. What is the differential diagnosis?
2. What other questions would you ask this patient?

Additional information: the patient follows a good lens care regimen. She does hot tub with her lenses, but denies any trauma or previous episodes or infections. She is told to stop the Viroptic, refrain from wearing her lenses, and use nonpreserved lubricating drops every 2 hours. She returns 1 week later, and on exam her visual acuity is 20/20 OD and 20/50 OS; there is moderate conjunctival injection, a central corneal infiltrate with mild edema and no epithelial defect, and 1+ anterior chamber cells. The appearance of the corneal infiltrate is shown:

3. What is the diagnosis?
4. What stains and culture media are used to identify this organism?
5. What is the appropriate management of this patient?
6. The patient requires a corneal transplant; what is the prognosis?

1. HSV keratitis, Viroptic toxicity, *Acanthamoeba* keratitis.

2. What is her lens care regimen? Does she use homemade solutions? Any recent swimming or hot tubbing with the contacts? Any recent trauma to the eye? Has she ever had a similar episode or eye infection in the past?

3. *Acanthamoeba* keratitis.

4. Stains: Giemsa and Calcofluor white. Culture media: nonnutrient agar with *E. coli* overgrowth.

5. Topical treatment with a combination of antibacterial, antifungal, and antiparasitic agents for months: neomycin or paromomycin; miconazole or clotrimazole (and oral voriconazole, ketoconazole or itraconazole); Brolene or hexamidine; and Baquacil or chlorhexidine. A topical cycloplegic drop should also be prescribed, and epithelial débridement should be considered.

6. There is a 30% recurrence rate after PK.

A 38-year-old woman complains of recurrent eye inflammation over the past 6 months. She says topical antibiotic drops prescribed by her internist for conjunctivitis have helped, but her eyes still feel uncomfortable and swollen.

1. What condition does the photo demonstrate that can be associated with her symptoms?

Additional information: inspection of her eyelids reveals the following:

2. Describe the findings.
3. What is the diagnosis?
4. What are the types of blepharitis?
5. What are the signs of anterior blepharitis?
6. What are the treatment options for this patient?

1. Her facial appearance shows acne rosacea; ocular involvement occurs in >50%.

2. Inflamed, obstructed Meibomian glands; pouting Meibomian gland orifices; thickened, opaque meibum; and telangiectasia of the lid margin.

3. Meibomian gland dysfunction (MGD; posterior blepharitis, meibomitis).

4. Blepharitis is often classified as anterior (seborrheic or staphylococcal), posterior (MGD), and angular (associated with *Moraxella*).

5. Debris at the base of the eyelashes (scurf and collarettes), lid margin erythema, loss of eyelashes, conjunctival injection; sequelae include pannus, phlyctenules, corneal infiltrates and ulcers.

6. Treatment for MGD includes lid hygiene (hot compresses, lid massage and lid scrubs), oral doxycycline or minocycline, oral fish oil (omega-3 fatty acids), topical azithromycin, topical steroids, topical cyclosporine, lubricating drops (for associated dry eye), LipiFlow, IPL therapy, and intraductal Meibomian gland probing. The patient may also benefit from treatment for acne rosacea.

A 52-year-old woman is seen for a routine eye exam and noted to have the finding shown in the photo.

1. What is the diagnosis?

2. What is the etiology?

3. What symptoms would the patient likely have?

4. What other substances can deposit in the cornea?

1. Cornea verticillata (vortex keratopathy).

2. Fabry's disease (X-linked recessive; including female carriers) and medications (most notably amiodarone; also chloroquine, indomethacin, ibuprofen, naproxen, chlorpromazine, suramin, clofazamine, tamoxifen).

3. None; the deposits are asymptomatic.

4. Calcium (band keratopathy), copper (chalcosis, Wilson's disease), cysteine (cystinosis), iron (from tears or hyphema), ink (corneal tattoo), lipid/cholesterol (dyslipoproteinemias), melanin, tyrosine (tyrosinemia), urate (gout), other medications (epinephrine (topical), ciprofloxacin (topical q1-2 hour), silver (argyrosis), gold (chrysiasis), mercury (topical drop preservative), thorazine/stelazine).

A 73-year-old man complains of redness and tearing from his left eye.

1. What is the diagnosis?
2. What are the possible etiologies?
3. How would you work up this patient?
4. What is the treatment?

1. Ectropion.

2. Cicatricial, congenital, inflammatory, involutional, mechanical, and paralytic.

3. Additional history about eye surgery, trauma, burns, infection or facial droop (ie, Bell's palsy) should be obtained to help determine the cause of the ectropion. Examination of the lids and adnexae with respect to orbicularis function, lateral canthal tendon laxity (snap-back test, distraction test), herniated fat, and scarring will also aid in establishing the etiology. Additionally, it is important to carefully inspect the inferior tarsal and bulbar conjunctiva and the cornea for signs of dryness/inflammation from exposure.

4. Ectropion-related corneal and conjunctival exposure is treated with topical lubrication (artificial tears, gel, and ointment). Treatment of the eyelid malposition depends on the etiology:

   Cicatricial: cicatrix revision/relaxation, horizontal tightening, may require vertical lengthening with full-thickness graft.

   Congenital: same as cicatricial but usually not required.

   Inflammatory: treat underlying condition.

   Involutional: horizontal shortening (lateral tarsal strip), lateral canthoplasty, repair of lower eyelid retractors.

   Mechanical: treat underlying condition.

   Paralytic: usually resolves within 6 months (Bell's palsy), otherwise lateral tarsorrhaphy, horizontal tightening, hard palate mucosal graft for lower eyelid elevation, upper eyelid gold weight implantation to improve closure.

A 27-year-old man complains of acute eye pain, redness, and decreased vision for 3 days.

1. What abnormality is shown, and what is the most likely diagnosis?

2. What is the differential diagnosis of dendritic keratitis?

3. What is the treatment of HSV epithelial keratitis?

4. What is the HEDS study recommendation for treatment of HSV stromal keratitis?

5. What are the complications of HSV keratitis?

6. How else can this disease manifest in the eye?

1. Corneal dendrite; HSV epithelial keratitis.

2. Herpes simplex, herpes zoster, Acanthamoeba, tyrosinemia, Thygeson's superficial punctate keratitis, healing epithelial defect.

3. Topical antiviral (Zirgan has less corneal toxicity than Viroptic), consider oral antiviral (acyclovir, famciclovir, or valacyclovir). For recurrent HSV keratitis, consider prophylaxis with long-term oral antiviral.

4. Treatment with topical steroids and Viroptic is better than Viroptic alone, and concomitant oral acyclovir has no additional benefit for the treatment of stromal keratitis. However, oral acyclovir reduces the risk of recurrent ocular disease, especially for patients with stromal keratitis.

5. Uveitis, glaucoma, episcleritis, scleritis, corneal scarring and neovascularization, corneal perforation, iris atrophy, and punctal stenosis (from topical antiviral drugs).

6. In addition to primary epithelial keratitis and various forms of recurrent keratitis, HSV may also cause vesicular blepharitis, follicular conjunctivitis, uveitis, and retinitis.

A 61-year-old woman complains that her eyes water. She has difficulty reading for more than 20 minutes at a time because of tearing and blurry vision, and at other times her eyes burn.

1. How would you evaluate this patient?
2. What specific tests are helpful?

Additional information: upon further questioning she reports chronic eye irritation for years, worse at the end of the day and after long periods of working on the computer. She can no longer wear contact lenses comfortably and only gets temporary relief from lubricating drops, which she uses several times a day. She denies any ocular surgery or trauma and does not have any allergies. Her medical history is notable for hypertension for which she takes hydrochlorothiazide. Slit lamp exam shows:

3. How is dry eye classified?
4. What are the treatment options?

1. Tearing, burning, and blurred vision are common symptoms of dry eye disease, so it is important to differentiate from other ocular surface disorders (blepharitis, allergic conjunctivitis) and other causes of tearing (ie, eyelid malposition, punctal stenosis, nasolacrimal duct obstruction, conjunctivochalasis). The correct diagnosis is determined with a detailed history of her symptoms (quality, timing, duration, exacerbating and ameliorating factors; consider using a questionnaire [OSDI, DEQ, NEI VFQ-25, McMonnies]), previous treatment, past ocular (particularly contact lens wear and previous eye or lid surgery) and medical (especially autoimmune disorders) histories, and medications, as well as a careful exam of the lids, lashes, conjunctiva, cornea, and tear film.

2. Surface staining with vital dyes (lissamine green or rose bengal for conjunctiva and cornea, fluorescein for cornea), height of tear meniscus, tear breakup time, tear production (Schirmer test, phenol red thread test), tear osmolarity, tear matrix metalloproteinase (MMP)-9 level; also tear lactoferrin and lysozyme levels and impression cytology. Corneal topography or keratometry may show dry spots and irregularity.

3. Dry eye disease (DED) is usually classified as aqueous deficient (abnormal lacrimal gland function resulting in decreased tear production) or evaporative (normal lacrimal gland function but increased tear evaporation because of lipid or mucin deficiency). Most cases of dry eye are multifactorial, and approximately 86% of patients with dry eye have signs of MGD.

    Aqueous deficient: Sjogren syndrome and nonSjogren syndrome (primary and secondary lacrimal gland deficiencies, obstruction of lacrimal duct, neurosecretory block (sensory or motor)).

    Evaporative: intrinsic (MGD, lid/globe abnormalities, reduced blinking, medications) and extrinsic (vitamin A deficiency, topical drugs, contact lens wear, cicatrizing or allergic conjunctivitis).

    The DEWS report classified DED by severity level (based on symptoms and signs) and recommended treatments accordingly:
    Level 1: mild symptoms, mild conjunctival signs, no staining
    Level 2: moderate symptoms, tear film and visual signs, conjunctival staining, mild corneal staining
    Level 3: severe symptoms, marked corneal staining, filamentary keratitis
    Level 4: extremely severe symptoms, severe corneal staining, corneal erosions, conjunctival scarring

4. Treatments include: lubrication (artificial tears, gels, ointments, lacrisert), topical cyclosporine (Restasis), topical lifitegrast (Xiidra), topical steroids, punctal occlusion, oral fish oil supplements (omega-3 fatty acids), humidifier. More severe cases may require autologous serum drops, bandage contact lens, Boston ocular surface prosthesis (PROSE lens), moisture chamber goggles, lid taping at bedtime, tarsorraphy. It is also important to reduce or eliminate associated factors and to treat any underlying conditions.

A 72-year-old woman 3 months status post uncomplicated cataract surgery in the left eye complains of blurry vision for 2 weeks. The cornea is clear, there is a mild anterior chamber reaction, and the IOL is centered in the bag.

1. What is the differential diagnosis?

2. What are the characteristic signs of chronic endophthalmitis?

3. What is the most likely causative organism?

4. How would you confirm the diagnosis?

Additional information: the culture is positive for P. acnes.

5. What is the treatment?

1. Intraocular inflammation due to rebound iritis, retained lens material, or delayed-onset/chronic endophthalmitis.

2. Posterior capsular plaque, iritis, keratic precipitates, may have keratitis, hypopyon, mild vitritis, and cystoid macular edema.

3. *Propionibacterium acnes*, coagulase-negative *Staphylococcus*, or fungi (*Candida* or *Aspergillus*). Other rarer organisms include *Actinomycetes* and *Nocardia*.

4. Anterior chamber tap for culture and smear.

5. *P. acnes* endophthalmitis is treated with intraocular vancomycin and topical steroids. It usually also requires a vitrectomy, injection of vancomycin into the capsular bag, partial or total capsulectomy, and IOL removal or exchange.

An 84-year-old man with aphakia OD and pseudophakia OS wears a rigid gas permeable contact lens OD, which gives him 20/25 vision. However, he finds it increasingly difficult to insert and remove the contact lens, so he is interested in surgery.

1. What are the secondary IOL options?
2. How would you determine where to place the lens?
3. What other findings are important to note for planning the surgical procedure?

Additional information: the patient has a large corneoscleral wound superiorly with thinning. The cornea is clear without guttata, there is a sector iridectomy superiorly, and some peripheral capsule is visible. The angle is open with scattered peripheral anterior synechiae (PAS), and there is a small knuckle of vitreous prolapsing into the anterior chamber.

4. What surgical technique would you recommend?
5. What are the disadvantages of a scleral-sutured IOL?

1. Secondary IOL in the bag, sulcus (with or without suture fixation to the iris or sclera), iris-fixated, or anterior chamber.

2. Placement depends on anatomic factors, health of the eye, patient's general health, and surgeon preference/comfort. It is important to assess the status of the cornea, angle, any remaining lens capsule, macula, peripheral retina, and optic nerve. Can the patient tolerate a lengthy procedure? Is the patient on anticoagulation?

3. Location of previous cataract wound, presence of iridectomy, posterior synechiae to capsule, amount and stability of any capsule, and vitreous in the anterior chamber.

4. A sulcus lens, possibly with suture support or an iris-fixated IOL is the only choice since there is no intact capsule for in the bag placement and there are PAS, which is a contraindication for an anterior chamber IOL. Because of the thinning at the superior limbus from the previous surgical wound, a temporal incision is preferred for this case. An anterior vitrectomy must be performed first to clear all vitreous anterior to the capsular plane. For unsutured sulcus placement, it is necessary to assess the remaining capsule for adequacy of supporting a posterior chamber IOL. If support appears to be sufficient, then a foldable three-piece or rigid one-piece IOL can be placed in the sulcus. The IOL stability must be tested by decentering the IOL in various meridians and observing for spontaneous recentration. If the IOL is not stable, then suture fixation to the iris may be performed. If it initially appears that capsular support is inadequate, then the IOL can be sutured to the iris or to the sclera. Alternatively, an iris-fixated (iris-claw) lens can be used. After placement of the IOL, the sector iridectomy can be repaired with several McCannel sutures. These sutures can be tied externally or internally using the Siepser technique.

5. It is technically more difficult, takes more time, and requires a thorough anterior vitrectomy. The main risks are long-term stability and damage to uveal tissue. Other complications include IOL tilt, IOL decentration, pigment dispersion, uveitis, intraocular hemorrhage (hyphema, vitreous hemorrhage, choroidal hemorrhage), suture exposure or erosion, endophthalmitis, CME, and retinal detachment. Numerous techniques have been developed to minimize these risks.

A 78-year-old man has a visually significant cataract and desires surgery. On exam, he dilates poorly and his lens appearance is seen in the photo.

1. What condition does he have and what other ocular problems are associated with it?
2. What other history would be helpful?

Additional information: the patient has a history of increased IOP, but has not been treated. He has an enlarged prostate and has taken tamsulosin (Flomax) for 2 years.

3. What would you pay particular attention to on exam?
4. What specific risks does this patient have with respect to cataract surgery?
5. What is IFIS?
6. How is IFIS managed?

1. Pseudoexfoliation syndrome (PXS), which is associated with angle closure, ectopia lentis, ocular hypertension and glaucoma (PXG).

2. What is his past ocular and medical history? Does he have any other ocular problems or has he been treated for any eye conditions? What medications does he take? Specifically, does he take medicine for his prostate or blood pressure?

3. Gonioscopy, diameter of dilated pupil, iridodonesis, phacodonesis, corneal pachymetry, IOP, and optic nerve appearance.

4. There is an increased risk of complications due to both the pseudoexfoliation (weak zonules) and Flomax (IFIS [intraoperative floppy iris syndrome]). He should be warned that these conditions increase the chance of complications such as posterior capsular rupture, vitreous loss, retained lens fragments, alternate lens placement, late lens dislocation, iris damage, and misshapen pupil. He should also be informed that PXS increases his risk for glaucoma (PXG) in the future, even if the lens is removed.

5. IFIS is a condition characterized by a variable degree of poor pupillary dilation, and floppy/atonic iris that billows, prolapses, and becomes miotic during surgery.

6. Mild forms may respond to preoperative topical atropine and intraocular preservative-free epinephrine. More severe forms require iris stabilization with one or more of the following: Healon 5, pupil expanders (Malyugin ring, Graether ring, I-ring, etc.), iris hooks, and low-flow fluidics during phacoemulsification.

A 52-year-old asymptomatic woman comes in for a complete eye exam. An anterior segment exam shows the finding in the photo. A posterior segment exam shows mild attenuation of the retinal vasculature and diffuse pigmentary changes in both eyes.

1. What questions would you ask her?

Additional information: she reports a few episodes of "conjunctivitis" for which she was given antibiotic and steroid drops. Cultures or additional workup were not performed. Her past medical history is positive for Chlamydia at age 28 and hypercholesterolemia.

2. What would you do next?

Additional information: the tests are negative except for a positive VDRL and FTA-ABS.

3. What treatment would you prescribe and why?
4. What is the organism?
5. What other ocular findings occur in this disease?
6. What are the systemic signs of congenital syphilis?

1. Does she have any past ocular history (disease, infection, trauma)? Has she ever had an episode of a red eye with blurry vision or photophobia? Is there any past medical history, specifically arthritis, autoimmune disorders, or infectious disease? Has she ever had a sexually transmitted disease?

2. The patient has had bilateral uveitis and requires a workup including CBC, RF, ANA, ACE, VDRL or RPR, FTA-ABS or MHA-TP, PPD and controls, and CXR.

3. Lumbar puncture to rule out neurosyphilis, and treat the patient and all sexual partners with systemic penicillin (or tetracycline if allergic to penicillin). Follow serum VDRL or RPR to monitor treatment efficacy.

4. *Treponema pallidum*, a spirochete.

5. Interstitial keratitis, uveitis, ectopia lentis, Argyll–Robertson pupil, chorioretinitis, and optic atrophy.

6. Saber shins, saddle nose, peg teeth, internal organ inflammation.

A 37-year-old man wants a new glasses prescription.

1. What finding is depicted in the photo?
2. What is the diagnosis?
3. What other findings would you expect to see?
4. What are the ocular associations?
5. If this patient develops high IOP requiring treatment, what would you recommend?
6. What is the pathophysiology?
7. What is the mechanism of glaucoma?
8. What is the natural course of the condition?

1. Kruckenberg spindle.

2. Pigment dispersion syndrome (PDS) or pigmentary glaucoma (PG).

3. Heavily pigmented trabecular meshwork, radial midperipheral iris transillumination defects, pigment in iris furrows and anterior lens capsule, iridodonesis, may have increased IOP (IOP spikes with blurry vision and halos may occur from exercise or pupil dilation), optic nerve cupping, and visual field defects.

4. Myopia, lattice degeneration (20%), PG develops in up to 50% of patients with PDS.

5. PDS/PG tends to respond well to laser trabeculoplasty so this may be a better initial choice than using a topical medication (with associated side effects and cost) indefinitely. Miotics (ie, pilocarpine) minimize the iris–zonule touch.

6. Reverse pupillary block. The iris has a concave configuration with contact against the zonules. Iris movement causes pigment liberation from the posterior surface as it rubs against the underlying zonules during normal pupillary movement.

7. PG is a secondary open-angle glaucoma in which iris pigment obstructs the trabecular meshwork causing elevated IOP and optic nerve damage.

8. PDS usually burns itself out because once all the pigment has been liberated, there is no more to clog the trabecular meshwork and raise the IOP.

A 46-year-old woman complains that her distance vision has gotten worse over the past year and she has needed frequent changes in the left lens of her glasses.

1. What is the differential diagnosis?

Additional information: she has no past ocular or medical history and she does not take any medication.

2. If a routine ophthalmic exam appeared normal, what other ocular testing would you perform?

Additional information: further exam shows increased cylinder on refraction, normal corneal topography and gonioscopy, and a segmental cataract in the left eye.

3. What is the most likely diagnosis and what test would you use to confirm it?
4. This patient has a ciliary body melanoma. What other findings may occur?
5. What is the treatment?

1. The change in refractive error is due to induced myopia, hyperopia, or astigmatism, which can result from systemic or ocular conditions. The differential diagnosis is:

   Acquired myopia:
   Increased lens power: nuclear sclerotic cataract, change in lens position or shape (medication [miotics]), anterior lens dislocation, excessive accommodation), osmotic effect (diabetes, galactosemia, uremia, sulfonamides), anterior lenticonus.
   Increased corneal power: keratoconus, contact lens-induced corneal warpage, congenital glaucoma.
   Increased axial length: posterior staphyloma, after scleral buckle surgery, congenital glaucoma, retinopathy of prematurity.

   Acquired hyperopia:
   Decreased refractive power: lens change (posterior lens dislocation, aphakia, diabetes), drugs (chloroquine, phenothiazines, antihistamines, benzodiazepines), poor accommodation (tonic pupil, drugs, trauma), flattening of cornea (contact lens).
   Decreased effective axial length: retrobulbar tumor, choroidal tumor, central serous chorioretinopathy.

   Acquired astigmatism:
   Lid lesion (tumor, chalazion, ptosis), pterygium, limbal dermoid, corneal degenerations and ectasias, surgery (corneal, cataract), lenticular, ciliary body tumor.

2. Corneal topography, gonioscopy, UBM, OCT, B scan ultrasound.

3. Ciliary body tumor, which can be visualized with UBM, anterior segment OCT, or Scheimpflug imaging.

4. In addition to lenticular astigmatism and cataract, signs of CB melanoma include shallow anterior chamber, sentinel vessel, and extrascleral extension.

5. Depending on the extent of the tumor, treatment is with surgical excision, chemotherapy, radiation, or enucleation.

A 50-year-old man presents with a recurrence of acute anterior uveitis and reports multiple episodes over the past 15 years. Exam of the involved eye shows 20/40 vision, ciliary flush, 2+ anterior chamber cells and flare, hypopyon, fine keratic precipitates, and no vitreous cells.

1. What additional history would be helpful?

2. What other findings would you look for on exam?

3. What is the differential diagnosis?

Additional information: the patient has no significant past medical history. He denies ocular herpes. He has eczema and occasional back pain, and he takes NSAIDs as needed. He travels internationally several times a year. IOP and gonioscopy are normal.

4. What targeted workup would you order?

5. What disorders are associated with HLA-B27 iritis?

6. What is the treatment for this patient's acute iritis?

7. What are the possible complications of iritis?

1. Past medical history, medication history, and review of systems with attention to joint pain, skin changes/ rashes, infections, oral lesions, urethritis, genital ulcers, diarrhea, foreign travel, and conjunctivitis.

2. Increased IOP, corneal edema, corneal scarring, synechiae, iris color, iris atrophy, cataract, and cystoid macular edema.

3. The differential diagnosis of nongranulomatous iritis is idiopathic, HLA-B27 associated, Fuchs' heterochromic iridocyclitis, HSV, glaucomatocyclitic crisis (Posner–Schlossman syndrome), Lyme disease, Behçet's disease, drugs, and interstitial nephritis.

4. This patient most likely has iritis associated with HLA-B27, so a targeted approach would be to order HLA-B27, sacroiliac X-ray, CBC with differential, urinalysis, VDRL or RPR, and FTA-ABS or MHA-TP.

5. Ankylosing spondylitis, Reiter's syndrome, psoriatic arthritis, inflammatory bowel disease, and Whipple's disease.

6. Frequent topical steroids and cycloplegia.

7. Cataract, glaucoma, synechiae, band keratopathy, iris atrophy, cystoid macular edema.

A 61-year-old woman says that her blue eye is turning brown.

1. What is the differential diagnosis?

2. On clinical exam, how is a nevus differentiated from a melanoma?

3. If you suspect a melanoma, what tests may be helpful?

Additional information: the pathology shows:

4. What is the diagnosis?

5. What are the various presentations of this disease?

6. What is the treatment?

7. What is the prognosis?

1. A pigmented iris lesion could be a nevus, melanocytoma, melanoma, iris pigment epithelial tumor, or rarely metastasis (usually amelanotic).

2. An iris nevus can be distinguished from a melanoma by: size (<3 mm in diameter), thickness (<1 mm thick), and the absence of vascularity, ectropion uveae, secondary cataract, secondary glaucoma, and growth.

3. Iris fluorescein angiogram (a nevus has a filigree filling pattern that becomes hyperfluorescent early and leaks late or is angiographically silent, whereas a malignant melanoma has irregular vessels that fill late), and B-scan ultrasound or UBM to rule out ciliary body involvement. Transillumination may also be helpful.

4. Malignant melanoma (spindle cell).

5. An iris malignant melanoma may be diffuse (associated with heterochromia and secondary glaucoma), tapioca (dark tapioca appearance), ring-shaped, or localized. It may have feeder vessels, involve angle structures, cause sectoral cataract, hyphema, increased IOP, or glaucoma.

6. Treatment includes chemotherapy, radiation, complete surgical excision, and enucleation depending on the extent. The patient may need treatment of increased IOP.

7. The prognosis is good, with a mortality rate of less than 10% and overall risk of metastasis of 14%.

A 66-year-old hyperopic man with best-corrected visual acuity of 20/60 OD and 20/30 OS desires cataract surgery in both eyes.

1. What additional history and testing would you obtain to determine if he is a suitable candidate for surgery in the left eye?

2. What are the etiologies and symptoms associated with this type of cataract?

3. What are the medical indications for cataract surgery?

4. The patient is extremely anxious and wants general anesthesia for the phacoemulsification procedure. You decide to use monitored anesthesia care and a retrobulbar block. What are possible complications of a retrobulbar injection?

5. During surgery, the patient starts to cough. What complications can result from this?

6. During IOL implantation, a darkening of the red reflex is seen, the iris prolapses, and the IOL cannot be placed in the bag due to vitreous pressure. What is happening?

7. How would you treat this?

1. How does the reduced vision interfere with his daily activities and hobbies? Does he have sensitivity to light? Is he experiencing difficulty in dimmer lighting conditions or with glare/halos from lights? Does he notice difficulty in reading? Helpful tests to perform include glare testing, near vision, pinhole vision, slit-lamp exam with attention to the type, degree, and density of the lens opacity, and the quality of the view on fundus exam.

2. Nuclear sclerotic and cortical cataracts are most commonly associated with age, ultraviolet (UV-B) exposure, and smoking. Both types of cataracts result in decreased and blurry vision and reduced contrast and color sensitivity. Nuclear sclerosis typically produces a myopic shift and more difficulty with distance than with near vision, while cortical spokes and vacuoles are more likely to cause glare and polyopia.

3. Cataracts that are causing a secondary eye disorder (ie, phacolytic, phacomorphic, or lens-particle glaucoma) or are obstructing the view of the posterior pole to the extent that they are interfering with the adequate diagnosis and treatment of retinal or optic nerve disease (ie, diabetes, macular degeneration, glaucoma).

4. Central anesthesia, retrobulbar hemorrhage, globe penetration/perforation, strabismus (inferior rectus fibrosis or myotoxicity).

5. Shallow chamber, iris prolapse, choroidal effusion/hemorrhage.

6. Choroidal effusion or suprachoroidal hemorrhage.

7. Immediately close the incision, administer mannitol, consider sclerotomies to drain blood/fluid, monitor the IOP, and implant the IOL at a later time (hours to days).

A 33-year-old woman complains of double vision and a funny looking pupil in her left eye.

1. What is the differential diagnosis of monocular diplopia?

2. What condition do you suspect she has?

3. What are the characteristic findings of each disorder in this syndrome?

4. What is the pathophysiology?

5. How is this distinguished from the mesodermal dysgenesis syndromes?

6. What are the mesodermal dysgenesis syndromes and the findings of each?

1. Uncorrected refractive error, cataract, corneal pathology (irregular astigmatism from anterior basement membrane dystrophy, scar, or ectasia), iris hole(s), rarely macular pathology.

2. Iridocorneal endothelial (ICE) syndromes, specifically essential iris atrophy.

3. The three syndromes that comprise ICE have the common features of iris distortion, corneal edema, and secondary angle-closure glaucoma due to angle endothelialization and peripheral anterior synechiae formation. The specific findings of each syndrome are:

   Iris nevus (Cogan–Reese) syndrome: flattening and effacement of the iris stroma, pigmented iris nodules (pseudonevi) composed of normal iris cells that are bunched up from the overlying membrane, corectopia, and ectropion uveae.

   Chandler's syndrome: corneal edema often with normal IOP, and mild or no iris changes (minimal corectopia, iris atrophy, peripheral anterior synechiae).

   Essential iris atrophy (progressive iris atrophy): proliferating endothelium produces broad PAS, corectopia, ectropion uveae, and iris holes (stretch holes [area away from maximal pull of endothelial membrane is stretched so thin that holes develop] and melting holes [holes in areas without iris thinning due to iris ischemia]).

4. Abnormal corneal endothelium grows across the angle and iris, obstructs the trabecular meshwork, distorts the iris, and contracts around the iris stroma to form nodules.

5. ICE is a unilateral, nonhereditary, progressive abnormality of the corneal endothelium that is not associated with any systemic abnormalities. It most commonly affects middle-aged women.

   Mesodermal dysgenesis is bilateral, congenital, and hereditary.

6. Axenfeld's anomaly: posterior embryotoxon (anteriorly displaced Schwalbe's line) with iris processes to the scleral spur. Glaucoma develops in 50%:

   Alagille's syndrome: Axenfeld's plus pigmentary retinopathy, corectopia, esotropia, and systemic abnormalities (absent deep tendon reflexes, abnormal facies, pulmonic valvular stenosis, peripheral arterial stenosis, biliary hypoplasia, and skeletal abnormalities).

   Rieger's anomaly: Axenfeld's plus iris hypoplasia with holes. Glaucoma develops in 50%.

   Rieger's syndrome: Rieger's anomaly plus mental retardation and systemic abnormalities (dental, craniofacial, genitourinary, and skeletal).

   Peter's anomaly: central corneal leukoma (opacity due to defect in Descemet's membrane with absence of endothelium) with iris adhesions, may have cataract and develop glaucoma (50%), and is associated with cardiac, craniofacial, and skeletal abnormalities. It is usually sporadic and bilateral (80%).

A 68-year-old woman sees you 5 days after uncomplicated cataract surgery because her eye has become progressively red and painful with blurry vision.

1. What is the diagnosis?

2. What are the most common organisms?

3. What are the risk factors?

4. What steps have been shown to reduce the rate of endophthalmitis?

5. What are the characteristic findings?

6. What are the Endophthalmitis Vitrectomy Study (EVS) treatment recommendations?

7. How is toxic anterior segment syndrome (TASS) differentiated from acute endophthalmitis?

1. Acute postoperative endophthalmitis.

2. Ninety-four percent of acute postoperative endophthalmitis is caused by Gram-positive bacteria: coagulase-negative staphylococci (70%), *Staphylococcus aureus* (10%), *Streptococcus* species (11%). Only 6% is due to Gram-negative bacteria.

3. Complicated surgery (prolonged surgical time, disrupted posterior capsule, vitreous loss, wound leak, iris prolapse), blepharitis, diabetes, immunosuppression.

4. Preoperative: povidone-iodine on the ocular surface, barrier draping the eyelashes.
   Intraoperative: preservative-free antibiotics in irrigating solution (ie, vancomycin) or injected intracamerally at conclusion of surgery (ie, cefuroxime, vancomycin, or Vigamox).

5. Decreased visual acuity, lid edema, proptosis, conjunctival injection, chemosis, wound abscess, corneal edema, keratic precipitates, anterior chamber cells and flare, hypopyon, vitritis, poor red reflex, and may have positive Seidel test at wound.

6. Better than light perception (LP) vision: anterior chamber and vitreous tap to collect specimens for culture, and intravitreal antibiotics (vancomycin and ceftazidime or amikacin). Also treat with subconjunctival (vancomycin and cetfazidime or gentamicin) and topical (fortified vancomycin and ceftazidime) antibiotics and steroids, and a topical cycloplegic. Intravitreal steroids were not evaluated, and systemic antibiotics were not found to be beneficial.

   LP vision or worse: same as above but also perform pars plana vitrectomy.

7. TASS usually presents during the first 24–48 hours after surgery and is characterized by diffuse corneal edema, fibrin in the anterior chamber, low IOP (may be high later), and minimal or no vitritis. There is less redness, pain, and anterior chamber reaction than in endophthalmitis. Treatment is with topical steroids, consider topical NSAID, and may require ocular hypotensive medications if IOP becomes elevated.

A 42-year-old man reports gradual deterioration of vision in his left eye. The slit-lamp exam is notable for the finding shown here.

1. What are the possible etiologies?

2. What are the findings of Marfan's syndrome, Weill–Marchesani syndrome, homocystinuria, hyperlysinemia, and sulfite oxidase deficiency?

3. What symptoms may this patient have?

4. What are the treatment options?

5. What are the surgical techniques for lens extraction?

1. Ectopia lentis is caused by trauma, pseudoexfoliation syndrome, syphilis, Marfan's syndrome, Weill–Marchesani syndrome, Stickler's syndrome, Ehlers–Danlos syndrome, homocystinuria, hyperlysinemia, sulfite oxidase deficiency, aniridia, congenital glaucoma, megalocornea, hereditary ectopia lentis, and ectopia lentis et pupillae.

2. Marfan's syndrome: ectopia lentis (65%; usually superotemporal), glaucoma, keratoconus, cornea plana, axial myopia, retinal degeneration (salt and pepper fundus), retinal detachment, tall stature, disproportionate growth of extremities, arachnodactyly, joint laxity, pectus deformities, scoliosis, and increasing dilation of the ascending aorta with aortic insufficiency.

   Weill–Marchesani syndrome: ectopia lentis (usually inferiorly or anteriorly), microspherophakia, high lenticular myopia, cataract, microcornea, glaucoma (pupillary block), short stature, stubby fingers with broad hands, hearing defects, inflexible joints, mental retardation.

   Homocystinuria: bilateral ectopia lentis (90% usually inferonasal; 30% in infancy, 80% by age 15 years), enlarged globe, myopia, peripheral RPE degeneration, retinal detachment, early loss of accommodation, blonde hair, tall (marfinoid habitus with arachnodactyly), osteoporosis, fractures, seizures, mental retardation (50%), cardiomegaly, platelet abnormality with hypercoagulability (thromboembolism), 75% mortality by age 30 years.

   Hyperlysinemia: ectopia lentis, microspherophakia, and growth, motor and mental retardation.

   Sulfite oxidase deficiency: ectopia lentis (50%), enophthalmos, Brushfield's spots, seizures, mental retardation, frontal bossing.

3. Blurry vision due to induced refractive error, diplopia if the lens equator is in the visual axis, and may have symptoms of angle-closure glaucoma.

4. Glasses or contact lens for refractive error, miotics for diplopia, and consider lens extraction. Patients may require treatment of angle-closure glaucoma and any underlying disorder.

5. Phacoemulsification (with capsular support system and sutured capsular rings or ring segments for IOL placement in the bag, otherwise sulcus sutured IOL or anterior chamber IOL, and may require anterior vitrectomy) by anterior segment surgeon or lensectomy/vitrectomy by retinal surgeon depending on the degree of lens displacement and instability.

A 79-year-old woman with pseudoexfoliation syndrome status post uncomplicated cataract surgery 6 years ago notices increasing blurry vision after bumping her forehead on a towel rack in the bathroom 2 weeks ago.

1. What is the term for the finding demonstrated in the photo?

2. What are the etiologies?

3. How would you treat a subluxed IOL?

4. After IOL repositioning, the patient subsequently develops a visually significant posterior capsular opacification. What are the potential complications of a Nd:YAG laser posterior capsulotomy?

1. Sunset syndrome.

2. In the bag IOL: zonulolysis from trauma or any other condition that can cause ectopia lentis (see Case 108).

   Sulcus IOL: insufficient capsular support, inappropriate IOL (length too short for sulcus), capsular contraction with asymmetric haptic placement (1 in and 1 out of bag).

3. IOL repositioning or exchange. For repositioning, the haptics (or capsular tension ring if present) can be sewn to the iris or sclera using a variety of techniques. For exchange, depending on the adequacy of capsular support and the status of the anterior chamber, the lens options are a sulcus IOL (with or without suture fixation), an iris-fixated IOL, and an anterior chamber IOL.

4. The risks of this laser procedure are small but include increased IOP, iritis, IOL optic damage, IOL dislocation, posterior vitreous detachment, cystoid macular edema, corneal or retinal burn, retinal tear and detachment.

A 74-year-old man says he has pain in his left eye and forehead and blurry vision for 2 days.

1. What questions would you ask him?

Additional information: he reports a fever and malaise for the past day but no other GCA symptoms, and no previous episodes or past ocular history. The pain is lancinating and burning on the forehead and around the eye with eye ache and sensitivity to light. The eye exam is normal. Four days later he returns with the appearance shown in the photo.

2. What is the diagnosis?
3. What does a lesion on the tip of the nose mean?
4. What anterior segment eye findings would you look for?
5. How would you treat this patient?
6. If this patient was 37 years old, what additional history and testing would you obtain?
7. What are the possible complications?
8. What are the risk factors for PHN?
9. How can this complication be treated?

1. Has he experienced any other related symptoms or any neurologic symptoms? It is important to ask specifically about symptoms of giant cell arteritis: scalp tenderness (does it hurt when you brush your hair?), jaw claudication (does it hurt to chew food?), headaches, fever, unexpected weight loss, and joint pain (PMR). Has he had any previous episodes of eye pain and blurry vision? Did he experience loss of vision or just blurry vision? Is the blurry vision constant? Was the onset sudden or gradual? Is there any redness or discharge? Characterize the pain (sharp, dull, pressure, radiation, superficial, deep, constant, intermittent, duration, severity, etc.). Does he have any past ocular history?

2. Herpes zoster ophthalmicus (HZO; shingles).

3. Hutchinson's sign, which is a strong indicator of ocular involvement (nasociliary branch of the ophthalmic nerve [CN V_1]).

4. Conjunctivitis, keratitis (epithelial, stromal, or endothelial), iritis, and increased IOP.

5. A 7-day course of an oral antiviral starting within 72 hours of the rash reduces the time course and risk and severity of ocular involvement. Famciclovir or valacyclovir is preferable to acyclovir because of reduced risk of postherpetic neuralgia (PHN). Oral steroids also reduce the time course, duration and severity of acute pain, and the risk of PHN. Topical steroids and cycloplegic for iritis, and monitor IOP; may require low dose topical steroid indefinitely to prevent recurrence of uveitis. If corneal epithelial involvement occurs, then add a topical antibiotic. Prevention of herpes zoster is with vaccination in patients age 50 years or older (reduces incidence, severity, and duration of zoster, reduces incidence of pain, and reduces incidence of PHN).

6. Herpes zoster is rare in individuals younger than 40 years old unless they are immunocompromised, therefore a history of immunosuppression (cancer, HIV, etc.) should be determined and an HIV test considered.

7. Lid scarring (lagophthalmos, ectropion, entropion, trichiasis, madarosis), canalicular and punctal stenosis, symblepharon, exposure keratopathy, neurotrophic keratopathy, corneal scarring, scleritis, glaucoma, uveitis, iris atrophy and necrosis, cataract, cystoid macular edema, optic neuropathy, retinitis, cranial nerve palsies, orbital apex syndrome, and PHN.

8. Increasing age, severity of pain, severity of skin rash, presence of ocular involvement.

9. A variety of medications can be used to treat PHN including opioids, tricyclic antidepressants, gabapentin/pregabalin, cimetidine, carbamazepine, steroids, topical analgesics (lidocaine cream/gel, lidoderm patch, capsaicin cream), diphenhydramine (Benadryl), nerve blocks, and Botox injections.

A 51-year-old woman woke up with decreased vision and eye pain in the right eye. It is hard for her to open her eyes for the exam and she says she feels nauseous. She is allergic to penicillin and sulfa. The appearance of the anterior segment is shown in the photo.

1. What is the diagnosis?

2. What are the associations?

3. What exam findings would you expect to see?

4. How do you distinguish between appositional and synechial angle closure?

5. What provocative tests can be used to diagnose angle closure?

6. How would you treat this patient?

Additional information: when she returns 1 week after the laser iridotomy for a pressure check, her IOP is 30 mmHg, the iridotomy is patent, and gonioscopy reveals a narrow angle. Ultrasound biomicroscopy shows:

7. What is the diagnosis?

8. What is the pathophysiology of this condition?

9. How would you manage this?

229

1. Acute angle-closure glaucoma.

2. Anatomic features that predispose to angle closure are small anterior segment (hyperopia, nanophthalmos, microcornea, microphthalmos), anterior iris insertion (Eskimos, Asians, and African Americans), and shallow anterior chamber (large lens, plateau iris configuration, loose or subluxed lens, pseudoexfoliation syndrome).

3. Decreased vision, mid-dilated poorly reactive pupil with possible RAPD, conjunctival injection, corneal epithelial edema, markedly elevated IOP, shallow anterior chamber, closed angle, iris bombe, and possibly mild anterior chamber cells and flare, peripheral anterior synechiae, iris atrophy, glaukomflecken, optic nerve swelling and hyperemia.

4. Indentation gonioscopy with a 4- or 6-mirror lens (ie, Zeiss, Posner, Sussman). Indenting the cornea forces aqueous fluid peripherally toward the angle. The angle opens if closure is appositional and remains closed if closure is synechial.

5. Provocative tests include the prone test, dark-room test, prone dark-room test, and pharmacologic pupillary dilation. Testing is positive if the IOP rises >8 mmHg.

6. Acute angle closure is an ophthalmic emergency that requires immediate lowering of IOP. Treatment is with multiple topical hypotensive drops (ie, β-blocker, $α_2$-agonist, CAI, pilocarpine (may not be effective if IOP is >40 mmHg owing to sphincter ischemia and may cause the lens–iris diaphragm to move forward, worsening pupillary block)) and oral agents (CAI and hyperosmotic agent (isosorbide, glycerin [contraindicated in diabetics], or IV mannitol [risk of cardiovascular adverse effects])). CAIs should not be used in this patient because of her sulfa allergy. Also, a topical steroid is added for inflammation. Laser peripheral iridotomy is the definitive treatment and performed when the cornea is clear enough to provide an adequate view. Topical glycerin may be necessary to clear corneal edema. A surgical iridectomy may be necessary if a laser iridotomy cannot be performed.

7. Plateau-iris syndrome.

8. Plateau iris is characterized by anteriorly rotated ciliary processes, which push the peripheral iris forward resulting in a deep chamber centrally and flat iris contour with a sharp dropoff peripherally. Dilation causes the peripheral iris to fold into the angle and occlude the trabecular meshwork. There is no pupillary block.

9. Laser iridoplasty and miotics.

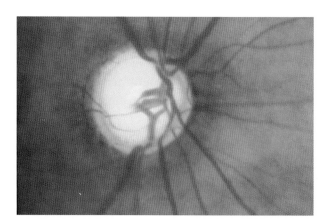

A 38-year-old man comes in for a complete eye exam. He says his vision has always been good and his last exam was more than 10 years ago. Exam shows 20/20 vision in both eyes, a peripheral posterior cortical/subcapsular cataract, and optic cupping in the right eye.

1. What additional history would be helpful?

2. How would you work up this patient?

Additional information: the patient says he was hit with a tennis ball in the right eye as a child and had blurry vision for a week or two but was not hospitalized and had no eye surgery. He denies any steroid use. IOP is 34 mmHg OD with normal corneal pachymetry. There is an inferior arcuate scotoma on HVF. Gonioscopy of the angle shows:

3. What finding is present?

4. What is the diagnosis?

5. What treatment would you recommend?

6. What surgical options are best for this type of glaucoma?

1. What is his past medical and ocular history? Is there a history of trauma, surgery, or steroid use? Does he take any medication? Does he have a family history of eye disease?

2. Slit-lamp exam with attention to signs of anterior segment injury (corneal scars, iris and angle tears, phacodonesis, cataract), check IOP, corneal pachymetry, gonioscopy, visual fields, optic nerve head photos, and nerve fiber layer analysis (OCT, confocal scanning laser ophthalmoscopy [HRT], scanning laser polarimetry [GDx]).

3. Angle recession, which is a tear in the ciliary body between the longitudinal and circular fibers of the ciliary muscle.

4. Angle recession glaucoma.

5. Initial treatment with topical medications. Laser trabeculoplasty has a poor effect on angle recession, so surgery is usually considered as the next step.

6. Trabeculectomy with antimetabolite or glaucoma drainage implant.

A 63-year-old man presents with decreased vision in the right eye.

1. What is the diagnosis?

2. What is the etiology?

3. What other findings would you look for on exam?

4. What is the treatment?

5. What are the complications of rubeosis?

6. What are the mechanism and treatment of NVG?

7. What is the treatment of hyphema?

8. What is an 8-ball hyphema?

9. What are the indications for anterior chamber washout?

1. Rubeosis (iris neovascularization).

2. Ocular ischemia, most commonly due to proliferative diabetic retinopathy, central retinal vein occlusion, and carotid occlusive disease. Rubeosis is also associated with anterior segment ischemia, chronic retinal detachment, tumors, sickle cell retinopathy, and chronic inflammation.

3. RAPD, increased IOP, corneal edema, angle neovascularization, retinal neovascularization/hemorrhages, or optic nerve cupping. Fluorescein angiogram may demonstrate retinal nonperfusion and neovascularization. Visual field testing may show glaucomatous defects.

4. Laser photocoagulation for retinal ischemia and possible peripheral cryotherapy. Treatment of increased IOP or glaucoma may be necessary.

5. Neovascular glaucoma (NVG) and hyphema. If the underlying cause is PDR, then vitreous hemorrhage and traction retinal detachment can occur.

6. NVG is a form of secondary angle-closure glaucoma. Neovascularization of the iris and angle results in occlusion of the trabecular meshwork. NVG usually requires a glaucoma drainage implant or cyclodestructive procedure to adequately control IOP.

7. Topical steroids and cycloplegic, may require treatment of increased IOP (do not use miotic agents or prostaglandin analogues, and avoid carbonic anhydrase inhibitors in patients with sickle cell disease), consider aminocaproic acid. Daily observation for the first 5 days to monitor the IOP and check for a rebleed. The patient should avoid aspirin-containing products, remain at bedrest, sleep with the head of the bed elevated, and protect the eye with a shield. Anterior chamber washout may be required.

8. A hyphema that has clotted and appears black or purple owing to impaired aqueous circulation and deoxygenated blood, which prevents resorption.

9. Anterior chamber washout is performed for corneal bloodstaining, uncontrolled elevated IOP, persistent blood clot, and rebleed.

An 80-year-old woman reports blurry vision and pain in her right eye for several months. Her past ocular history is significant for cataract surgery 20 years ago.

1. What is the diagnosis?
2. What are the other causes of bullous keratopathy?
3. How would you treat her?

1. Pseudophakic bullous keratopathy (PBK) due to a rigid anterior chamber IOL.

2. Corneal edema causing bullous keratopathy can also be due to aphakia, vitreocorneal touch, iridocorneal touch, severe or chronic keratitis, and breaks in Descemet's membrane (ie, birth trauma).

3. Temporary treatment of the corneal edema and any inflammation is with topical steroids and a cycloplegic. If the patient develops ruptured bullae, she should be treated with a topical antibiotic, lubrication, and bandage contact lens. A tarsorrhaphy may be necessary to heal a persistent epithelial defect. Anterior stromal puncture may help but the bullae often recur. Definitive treatment is IOL explantation or exchange, and corneal transplantation may also be required (endothelial or penetrating keratoplasty).

A 57-year-old woman with advanced glaucoma had a trabeculectomy last week. The appearance of her eye is shown.

1. What is the problem?
2. What findings would you look for on exam?
3. What is the differential diagnosis?
4. How does the anterior chamber appearance differ in angle-closure and malignant glaucoma?
5. You determine this patient has malignant glaucoma. How would you treat her?

1. Flat bleb.

2. IOP (decreased or increased), Seidel test, anterior chamber depth, and fundus appearance.

3. The differential diagnosis of a flat bleb depends on the IOP. If the IOP is low, then the cause is a bleb leak or choroidal detachment. If the IOP is high, then the cause is a suprachoroidal hemorrhage, pupillary block, or malignant glaucoma.

4. In angle closure the anterior chamber is deeper centrally than peripherally, whereas in malignant glaucoma the entire anterior chamber is shallow.

5. Medical management is with a topical cycloplegic and aqueous suppressants. If this does not resolve the condition, then Nd:YAG laser anterior vitreolysis (for pseudophakic or aphakic eyes) or vitrectomy (for phakic eyes) may be required.

A 29-year-old man complains of worsening right eye pain and blurred vision for the last week. He reports several similar episodes in the past but they all resolved within a few days. His past medical history is negative and he takes no medication.

1. What is the most likely diagnosis?

2. What other anterior segment signs might you find on exam?

Additional information: the patient has iris heterochromia and fine KP.

3. What is the diagnosis?

4. What are the eye findings specific to this form of anterior uveitis?

5. What is the etiology of iris heterochromia?

6. What is the treatment?

1. Iritis.

2. Ciliary injection, keratic precipitates (KP), anterior chamber cells and flare, posterior synechiae, altered IOP, iris atrophy, band keratopathy, cataract, cystoid macular edema.

3. Fuchs' heterochromic iridocyclitis.

4. Iris heterochromia (lighter in affected eye), diffuse iris atrophy, small white stellate KP, fine-angle vessels (may bleed during gonioscopy, cataract surgery, or paracentesis), no synechiae, and minimal anterior chamber reaction.

5. The etiology depends on whether the condition is congenital or acquired and the involved iris is lighter (hypochromic) or darker (hyperchromic):

   Congenital:

   Hypochromic: congenital Horner's syndrome, Waardenburg's syndrome, Hirschsprung's disease, Perry–Romberg hemifacial atrophy.
   Hyperchromic: ocular or oculodermal melanocytosis, iris pigment epithelium hamartoma.

   Acquired:

   Hypochromic: acquired Horner's syndrome, juvenile xanthogranuloma, iris metastatic carcinoma, Fuchs' heterochromic iridocyclitis, stromal atrophy (glaucoma or inflammation).
   Hyperchromic: siderosis, hemosiderosis, chalcosis, medication (topical prostaglandin analogues for glaucoma), iris nevus or melanoma, iridocorneal endothelial syndrome, iris neovascularization.

6. Topical cycloplegic and steroids (typically there is a poor response to topical steroids, so they should not be used for long-term treatment), and may require treatment of elevated IOP.

A 74-year-old woman undergoes complicated cataract surgery with posterior capsular rupture and retained lens fragment. On postoperative day 1, visual acuity is 20/60, there is mild conjunctival injection, moderate corneal edema, 2+ anterior chamber cells and flare, and a well-centered IOL in the sulcus.

1. How would you manage this patient?
2. What are the intraoperative signs of posterior capsular tear/rupture?
3. What surgical steps should be performed if a posterior capsular tear/rupture occurs?

1. The patient must be informed about the surgical complication, potential sequelae, and treatment plan. A dilated fundus exam is performed to identify retained lens material in the posterior segment and to examine the peripheral retina for tears (increased risk with vitreous loss).

   Management of retained material after cataract surgery depends upon the size, type (cortical vs. nuclear), and location (anterior segment vs. posterior segment) of the lens fragment(s). Nuclear material, even small chips, are generally poorly tolerated and should be removed promptly because they can induce severe intraocular inflammation with elevated IOP, corneal edema, and CME. Small pieces of cortex can be observed and may resorb over weeks to months with topical steroid treatment and careful observation. Cortex sequestered in the capsular bag rarely causes any complications.

   The inflammation is treated with topical steroids (a topical NSAID can also be used), and the patient may require treatment for elevated IOP. If a piece of nucleus is identified in the anterior chamber, surgical extraction by an anterior segment surgeon is indicated. Similarly, if nuclear material is present in the vitreous cavity, the patient should be referred to a retinal surgeon for evaluation and removal.

2. The signs depend upon when this complication occurs. During hydrodissection or phacoemulsification, there is usually a sudden deepening of the anterior chamber. The lens nucleus may shift or tilt or even dislocate into the posterior segment. Further phacoemulsification is accompanied by poor followability when vitreous is present in the anterior chamber. Posterior capsular tear/rupture occurring during subsequent steps (ie, I/A, lens insertion or manipulation) is usually directly visible as sudden posterior capsule striae followed by a hole or split in the capsule.

3. It is important to prevent collapse of the anterior chamber since this causes the vitreous to move forward and usually results in rupture of the anterior vitreous face. Therefore before removing an instrument from the main incision (ie, phaco or I/A tip), a dispersive viscoelastic should be injected through a side port incision to maintain the space and sequester any remaining nuclear material in the anterior chamber. A Sheets glide can be inserted to prevent nuclear material from falling posteriorly. Any vitreous prolapsing forward must be removed by performing a thorough anterior vitrectomy. Triamcinolone (Kenalog or Triesence) can be used to help visualize vitreous strands in the anterior chamber. The remaining nuclear pieces can be removed manually or with low-flow phaco settings (ie, lower the irrigation bottle height, reduce the aspiration flow rate and vacuum), and then the remaining cortex can be removed manually, with an I/A probe, or with a vitrector. Finally an IOL is inserted in an appropriate location, and its stability is checked to make sure it is secure. Depending on the type and position of the IOL, prior or after its insertion Miochol or Miostat can be injected to constrict the pupil. If the pupil does not become small and round, then vitreous may be prolapsing through the pupil or the IOL may be causing pupil ovalization or iris tuck, so additional manipulations may be required.

A 55-year-old man is found to have generous optic cups on routine eye exam.

1. What is the differential diagnosis?
2. What other history and exam findings are relevant?

Additional information: the patient is a low myope with no past ocular history. He denies previous trauma or steroid use, and there is no family history of glaucoma. His vision is 20/20 and the IOP is 18 mmHg OU, anterior segment exam is normal except for trace cortical vacuoles in the crystalline lens OU, and posterior segment exam shows large optic cups OU.

3. What testing would you perform?

Additional information: on subsequent exam, the IOP is 19 mmHg and corneal pachymetry measures 540 microns OU. There is a small hemorrhage present at the inferior disc margin OS. Humphrey visual field testing shows an enlarged blindspot OD and a small superior nasal step OS.

4. What is the diagnosis?
5. How would you manage this patient?

1. Physiologic cupping (usually myopic individuals), primary open-angle glaucoma (with large diurnal variations), "burned-out" secondary open-angle glaucoma (ie, pigmentary, uveitic, traumatic, steroid-induced glaucomas), chronic angle closure, normal tension glaucoma, neurologic disease (optic neuropathy, optic neuritis, chiasmal compressive lesions; usually have more pallor than cupping).

2. History of trauma, steroid use, uveitis, elevated intraocular pressure, family history of glaucoma, myopia. Exam findings suggestive of glaucomatous optic nerve damage in such a patient include Krukenburg spindle, keratic precipitates, iris transillumination defects, narrow angles, iris or angle tears, synechiae (peripheral anterior or posterior), elevated IOP, phacodonesis, PSC or traumatic cataract, nerve fiber layer defects, asymmetric cupping, splinter hemorrhage at nerve head.

3. Tonometry, corneal pachymetry, gonioscopy, visual fields, optic nerve head photos, and nerve fiber layer analysis; also consider performing a diurnal curve, optic nerve blood flow measurement (color Doppler imaging, laser Doppler flowmetry), ERG/VEP, and neurologic workup. Obtaining old ophthalmic records, if available, can also be helpful.

4. Normal tension glaucoma.

5. Treatment is to reduce intraocular pressure with medication, laser, or surgery. The Collaborative Normal Tension Glaucoma Study (CNTGS) demonstrated that lowering IOP by 30% or more reduced the rate of visual field loss; however, rate of progression without treatment is variable and usually slow (half of untreated patients had no progression after 5 years). NTG is more difficult to treat than POAG.

A 31-year-old man is noted to have ocular abnormalities on undilated slit lamp examination.

1. What findings are shown in the photo, and what is the diagnosis?
2. What is the etiology?
3. What are the associated findings?
4. What is the treatment?

1. Absence of iris and cataract; aniridia.

2. Aniridia is a rare, congenital defect in which the iris is absent bilaterally except for a small peripheral remnant. The defect is hereditary or sporadic and has been mapped to chromosome 11p13 (*PAX6* gene).

3. Aniridia causes photophobia and glare; findings include decreased vision, nystagmus, strabismus, and amblyopia. It is associated with lens opacities (up to 80%), glaucoma (up to 50%), ectopia lentis, corneal pannus, optic nerve, and foveal hypoplasia. There are three types of aniridia:

   AN 1: most common (85%), autosomal dominant, only ocular findings.

   AN 2: 13%, sporadic, associated with Wilms' tumor (Miller's syndrome and WAGR).

   AN 3: 2%, autosomal recessive, associated with mental retardation and cerebellar ataxia (Gillespie's syndrome) but not Wilms' tumor.

4. Treatment for photophobia and glare is a cosmetic/painted contact lens. An artificial iris implant can be inserted at the time of cataract surgery. Patients may require treatment for increased intraocular pressure and glaucoma.

A 48-year-old man complains of blurry vision in his right eye. His best-corrected visual acuity is 20/80 OD (with minimal improvement with pinhole) and 20/20 OS. Besides the finding shown in the photo, his eye exam is otherwise normal.

1. What is the diagnosis?
2. What are the causes and typical symptoms of this type of cataract?
3. What are the indications for cataract surgery?
4. Does this patient have any increased risk of complications from cataract surgery?

1. Posterior subcapsular cataract.

2. Posterior subcapsular cataracts are associated with aging, steroids, trauma, ionizing radiation, intraocular inflammation, diabetes, high myopia, retinitis pigmentosa, Refsum's disease, and atopic dermatitis. The characteristic symptoms are photophobia and glare especially from bright lights (ie, headlights while driving at night) and variable decreased vision typically worse at near than distance. Other symptoms of cataracts are reduced contrast and color sensitivity and sometimes monocular diplopia or polyopia.

3. The indication for cataract surgery is when the patient desires improved vision because of visual symptoms interfering with daily activities. Rarely, cataract surgery is performed for medical reasons such as the cataract is causing glaucoma or uveitis, or the cataract is interfering with the examination or treatment of another ocular disease (ie, macular degeneration, diabetic retinopathy, glaucoma) because the posterior segment cannot be adequately evaluated through the lens opacity.

4. There is no increased risk of a surgical complication unless the cataract is associated with trauma that has resulted in other ocular problems (ie, zonular weakness or dehiscence, vitreous prolapse, corneal scarring interfering with visualization of the lens).

An 87-year-old woman is seen urgently for increasing eye pain and loss of vision for several days.

1. What does the photo show?

2. What is the differential diagnosis?

3. What are the characteristics of each?

Additional information: exam shows visual acuity of light perception only, the IOP is 27 mmHg, the anterior chamber is deep, and there is a 3+ anterior chamber reaction with white flocculent material.

4. What is the treatment?

1. Mature cataract and conjunctival injection. The anterior chamber (depth and presence of inflammation) cannot be assessed from the photo.

2. Lens-induced glaucoma: phacolytic, phacomorphic, or lens particle.

3. Phacolytic: hypermature cataract leaks lens proteins through an intact capsule; trabecular meshwork obstructed by lens proteins and macrophages that ingest them.

   Phacomorphic: enlarged cataractous lens pushes the iris forward; the trabecular meshwork is obstructed by the iris (secondary angle-closure). Risk factors include hyperopia, short axial length, and shallow anterior chamber depth.

   Lens-particle: lens material from penetrating trauma or retained after cataract surgery causes inflammation (more than phacolytic and higher IOP, synechiae and inflammatory membranes); trabecular meshwork obstructed by lens material.

4. Topical treatment for inflammation (steroid and cycloplegic) and increased intraocular pressure should be initiated promptly. The definitive treatment for phacolytic glaucoma is urgent cataract surgery.

A 47-year-old woman reports blurry vision for several weeks.

1. What does the photo show?
2. What are the possible etiologies?
3. What other exam findings would you look for?
4. What other tests would be helpful and why?

Additional information: an ultrasound evaluation is performed. The B scan reveals a mass, and the A scan shows:

5. What is the most likely diagnosis and why?
6. How would you treat the patient?
7. What is the prognosis?

1. A dome-shaped, exudative retinal detachment (RD) without corrugation or surface membranes. In addition, there is no evidence of retinal traction. No obvious mass is seen in the picture.

2. The causes of an exudative retinal detachment include uveitis (VKH, sympathetic ophthalmia, pars planitis, posterior scleritis), tumors (especially retinal capillary hemangioma/von Hippel-Lindau disease, choroidal hemangioma, choroidal malignant melanoma), and hypertension. Other causes are glomerulonephritis, eclampsia/pre-eclampsia, hypothyroidism, Coats disease, scleritis, and central serous chorioretinopathy (CSC).

3. In general, exudative RDs are located inferiorly, display shifting fluid, and have a smooth appearance. The appearance of a smooth, retinal detachment behind the lens is almost pathognomonic for exudative RD. Chronic exudative RD can lead to neovascular glaucoma.

   It is important to perform a careful depressed dilated fundus examination to evaluate for peripheral retinal tears and breaks and rule out a rhegmatogenous retinal detachment; as well as evaluation for traction membranes to rule out a traction retinal detachment. Traction RDs are usually taut and immobile with a concave surface that does not extend to the ora serrata.

4. A fluorescein angiogram (FA) is useful to evaluate for tumors (intrinsic vasculature, feeder vessels) and vascular abnormalities. Indocyanine green angiography (ICG) is superior to FA to show intrinsic vascularity, hot spots, and washout phenomenon for tumors. A B-scan ultrasound should be performed to confirm the shifting fluid, evaluate choroidal thickness, and, more importantly, to evaluate for masses. An A-scan ultrasound is used to evaluate internal reflectivity if a mass is found. Optical coherence tomography (OCT) is useful to verify thickened choroid using enhanced depth imaging techniques in uveitic conditions, image the subretinal fluid and/or cystoid macular edema. Although rarely necessary, orbital imaging can be performed.

5. Choroidal hemangioma because of the high internal reflectivity.

6. The decision to treat is individualized based on extent of symptoms, loss of vision, and potential for visual recovery. The aim of treatment is to induce tumor atrophy with resolution of subretinal fluid and tumor-induced foveal distortion without destroying function of overlying retina. The goal is not to obliterate the tumor. Treatment options consist of laser photocoagulation (moderately intense, white reaction on the tumor surface to eliminate serous exudation), cryotherapy, ocular photodynamic therapy (PDT) with verteporfin (Visudyne) using standard treatment parameters, transpupillary thermotherapy, I-125 plaque brachytherapy, and low-dose external beam radiation therapy.

7. Visual loss can be progressive and irreversible when the fovea is involved in chronic cases. Poor visual acuity results can be expected despite resolution of fluid exudates from chronic macular edema and photoreceptor loss.

A 44-year-old man is worried about blurry vision in the right eye for the past 2 weeks.

1. What is the differential diagnosis?
2. What tests would be helpful?

Additional information: the FA shows:

3. What is demonstrated, and what is the diagnosis?
4. How would you manage this patient?

1. Central serous chorioretinopathy (CSC), inflammatory choroidal disorders (VKH syndrome), uveal effusion syndrome, optic nerve pit, choroidal tumor, vitelliform macular detachment, pigment epithelial detachment from other causes including choroidal neovascularization (CNV).

2. OCT to characterize the features present along with the obvious subretinal fluid including checking for macular schisis or optic nerve excavations seen with an optic nerve pit, a thickened choroid that is seen in VKH, central serous chorioretinopathy, and uveal effusion syndrome, or the characteristic OCT appearance of vitelliform lesions. A fluorescein angiogram (FA) would be useful to rule out choroidal neovascularization (although rare in this age group) and to visualize the hyperfluorescence early with late pooling of a pigment epithelial detachment and the subretinal fluid. If both these tests fail to determine the diagnosis, indocyanine green angiography (ICG) can show hyperfluorescence with late staining in CSC, vascularity with tumors, and rule out CNV. OCT angiography (OCTA) can be useful to also rule out CNV.

3. The FA shows "smoke-stack" leakage into the pigment epithelial detachment characteristic of CSC; however, this classic appearance is seen in only about 10% of cases.

4. Observation initially since most cases resolve spontaneously over 6 weeks. Off-label, anti-mineralocorticoid oral therapy (spironolactone or eplenerone), off-label rifampin, laser treatment or verteporfin (Visudyne) ocular photodynamic therapy (PDT) can be considered for patients who require more rapid visual recovery because of occupational reasons, poor vision in the fellow eye due to CSC, no resolution of fluid after several months, recurrent episodes with poor vision, or in severe forms of CSC. Treatment reduces the duration of symptoms but does not affect the final visual acuity.

A 49-year-old man complains of acute eye pain with decreased vision and photophobia.

1. What does the photo demonstrate?
2. What is the differential diagnosis?
3. What other findings would you look for on exam?
4. What lab tests would be helpful?

Additional information: the anterior chamber PCR is positive for HSV, and the HIV test is negative.

5. What is the diagnosis?
6. What is the treatment?
7. What are the potential complications?

1. A well-defined area of retinal necrosis with retinal whitening and intraretinal hemorrhages.

2. Acute retinal necrosis, progressive outer retinal necrosis (PORN), syphilis, cytomegalovirus retinitis, toxoplasmosis, sclopoteria, lymphoma, sarcoidosis, hemorrhagic occlusive retinal vasculitis (HORV; associated with intraocular vancomycin), and aminoglycoside toxicity.

3. Evidence of granulomatous anterior uveitis, vitritis, and retinal vasculitis.

4. PCR testing of intraocular fluid is the most precise method to determine the cause of the viral retinitis: herpes zoster virus (HZV), herpes simplex virus (HSV), or, rarely, cytomegalovirus (CMV). Alternatively, blood testing for HZV and HSV (type 1 and 2) immunoglobulin G and M titers can be performed. The immune status should be obtained to verify whether the patient is immunocompetent because it is important to differentiate ARN from PORN, which occurs in immunocompromised patients with minimal inflammation and vasculitis.

5. Acute retinal necrosis.

6. Immediately treat with antivirals since any delay in therapy can cause a dramatic increase in the retinitis. Typically, systemic acyclovir (IV until resolution of the retinitis then oral for 1–2 months); alternatively, if the lesions are more peripheral then use oral therapy with valacyclovir instead of IV therapy. Ganciclovir is an alternative. It is important to follow blood urea nitrogen (BUN) and creatinine levels for nephrotoxicity. Both oral and topical steroids can be started after the patient begins to respond to prevent inflammatory complications. Also treat with intravitreal foscarnet, follow closely for signs of regression, and if none seen additional injections may be required.

7. Patients with ARN are at high risk of developing rhegmatogenous retinal detachments with numerous holes and giant tears due to retinal necrosis. In addition, very careful observation of the fellow eye is important to rule out involvement.

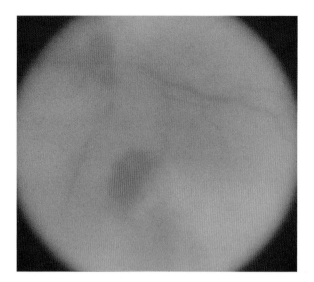

A 65-year-old man presents with blurred vision and floaters in both eyes for several months. On exam, his eyes are white and quiet, and there are bilateral dense sheets of vitreous cells. He says he has been treated by an outside doctor with topical steroids with no response.

1. What additional history would you want to know?
2. What is the differential diagnosis?
3. What tests would you perform?

Additional information: the pathology from a vitreous biopsy shows:

4. What is the diagnosis?
5. How would you treat this patient?
6. What additional testing should be performed?
7. What is the prognosis?

1. Has he had any unexplained fevers and chills, night sweats, fatigue, headaches, or weight loss? What is the past medical history, especially any cancer history? Is there any lymphadenopathy (especially cervical and supraclavicular), or any CNS symptoms?

2. Anything that produces a chronic vitritis including infectious and noninfectious uveitis such as birdshot chorioretinopathy, pars planitis, toxoplasmosis, syphilis, sarcoidosis, multifocal choroiditis, acute posterior multifocal placoid pigment epitheliopathy, Behçets disease, tuberculosis, and acute retinal necrosis; however, for a patient in this age group with these signs, primary intraocular lymphoma (PIOL) is of greatest concern.

3. Since PIOL is a masquerade syndrome, complete laboratory testing to rule out uveitis entities should be done including CBC, ESR, angiotensin-converting enzyme level, HLA-B 27 and 51, ANA test, and VDRL or RPR, FTA-ABS or MHA-TP testing. For additional testing paradigm see Case 126.

   With negative laboratory testing, a thorough neurological evaluation should be performed in search of CNS involvement including magnetic resonance imaging (MRI) of the brain and lumbar puncture for CNS cytology. If both are negative then a diagnostic pars plana vitrectomy should be performed. An undilute vitreous biopsy (approximately 1 cc) should be sent for cytology, flow-cytometry analysis for B- and T-cell markers and kappa/lambda light chains. Other ancillary tests include the measurement of IL-6 and IL-10 (high IL-10 and high ratio of IL-10 to IL-6 are suggestive of intraocular lymphoma).

4. Diffuse large B-cell non-Hodgkin's lymphoma.

5. The treatment of primary intraocular lymphoma is still controversial and includes intravitreal methotrexate and/or rituximab; and orbital radiation in cases without any CNS involvement. However, the majority of patients do develop CNS involvement, so most oncologists treat with chemotherapy with blood–brain barrier disruption or high-dose systemic methotrexate.

6. A complete metastatic survey (imaging studies of the chest and abdomen) and bone marrow biopsy.

7. 60–80% will develop CNS lymphoma within a mean of 29 months. The prognosis is poor if there is brain involvement.

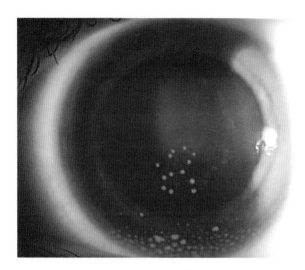

A 42-year-old woman reports pain, photophobia, redness, and decreased vision for 4 days. She recalls having had a similar episode several years ago.

1. What finding is shown, and what is the diagnosis?
2. What is the differential diagnosis?
3. What other findings may be present?
4. How would you work up a patient with granulomatous uveitis?

Additional information: the appearance of her retina is shown.

5. What is the diagnosis?
6. What is the treatment?

1. This patient has large mutton-fat keratic precipitates (KP), which is a sign of granulomatous uveitis.

2. Syphilis, tuberculosis, leprosy, brucellosis, toxoplasmosis, *P. acnes* endophthalmitis, fungal infection (*Cryptococcus*, *Aspergillus*), HIV, sarcoidosis, VKH syndrome, sympathetic ophthalmia, and a phacoanaphylactic reaction.

3. Ciliary injection, anterior chamber cells and flare, hypopyon, iris nodules, rubeosis, synechiae, increased or decreased IOP, cataract, pars planitis, optic nerve hyperemia, chorioretinitis, periphlebitis, and cystoid macular edema.

4. A basic battery of lab tests is recommended to determine the cause of granulomatous uveitis in a patient with a negative history, review of systems, and medical examination. This includes complete blood count (CBC) with differential, erythrocyte sedimentation rate (ESR), Venereal Disease Research Laboratory (VDRL; syphilis) or rapid plasma reagin (RPR; syphilis), treponemal antibody absorption test (FTA-ABS; syphilis) or microhemagglutination assay for treponema pallidum (MHA-TP; syphilis), ELISA or indirect immunofluorescence assay (IFA) for toxoplasma IgM and IgG titers, angiotensin-converting enzyme (ACE; sarcoidosis), lysozyme.

    Other labs tests can be ordered according to the patient's history including antinuclear antibody (ANA), rheumatoid factor (RF; juvenile rheumatoid arthritis), ELISA for Lyme immunoglobulin M (IgM) and immunoglobulin G (IgG), HIV antibody test, chest radiographs or CT scan (sarcoidosis, tuberculosis), sacroiliac radiographs (ankylosing spondylitis), and urinalysis.

    Special diagnostic lab tests can also be considered if the diagnosis is still unclear including HLA typing (HLA-A29: Birdshot chorioretinopathy), in the presence of vasculitis: ANCA (Wegener's granulomatosis, polyarteritis nodosa), Raji cell and C1q binding assays for circulating immune complexes (SLE, systemic vasculitides), complement proteins: C3, C4, total complement (SLE, cryoglobulinemia, glomerulonephritis), and soluble IL-2 receptor.

5. Toxoplasmosis chorioretinitis.

6. Topical steroids and cycloplegic are prescribed to treat the anterior inflammation. Systemic steroids are added for posterior pole lesions or those with intense inflammation.

    Small peripheral lesions may be observed since they often heal spontaneously especially in immunocompetent individuals. If a patient has decreased vision, moderate to severe vitreous inflammation, or lesions that threaten the macula, papillomacular bundle, or optic nerve he/she should be treated for 4–6 weeks with antibiotics that kill tachyzoites in the retina (note: they do not affect cysts). Most patients respond well to trimethoprim-sulfamethoxazole (Bactrim). For aggressive lesions or posterior pole lesions, triple therapy can be considered with pyrimethamine (Daraprim), folinic acid (leucovorin), and one of the following: sulfadiazine, clindamycin, clarithromycin, azithromycin, or atovaquone. Immunocompromised patients and high-risk patients may require prophylactic treatment.

A 38-year-old man with no previous ocular history reports irritation of his right eye after doing some work around the house. On exam, the patient has 20/20 vision and normal intraocular pressure. The appearance of the anterior segment is shown above.

1. What abnormality is present, and what is the likely cause?
2. How would you work up this patient?
3. How are foreign bodies classified?
4. What findings are seen in chalcosis and siderosis?
5. How would you treat this patient?

1. Iris defect due to an intraocular foreign body (IOFB).

2. Ask a detailed history about the type of work he was performing (ie, hammering, sawing, power tools)? Did he wear eye protection? Did he feel something hit or poke his eye?

   Obtain an orbital CT or X-ray to identify any intraocular foreign body (not an MRI if a metallic IOFB is suspected).

3. *Inert*: do not require removal (ie, glass, plastic, sand, stone, ceramic, gold, platinum, silver, aluminum).

   Reactive: cause inflammation/toxicity and must be removed (ie, copper [≥85% causes severe endophthalmitis, <85% causes chalcosis, <70% is relatively inert], iron [siderosis], wood/plant material [significant inflammation and higher risk of endophthalmitis]).

4. *Chalcosis*: mild intraocular inflammation, deposition of copper in the anterior lens capsule (sunflower cataract) and Descemet's membrane (Kayser–Fleisher ring), and retinal degeneration. The iris may become green and the pupil sluggishly reactive to light.

   Siderosis: iris heterochromia (hyperchromic on involved side), mid-dilated minimally reactive pupil, lens discoloration (brown-orange dots from iron deposition in lens epithelium, generalized yellowing from involvement of cortex), vitritis, pigmentary RPE degeneration with sclerosis of vessels, retinal thinning, and atrophy. In both diseases, the ERG is reduced or even absent.

5. Surgical exploration and repair with removal of any reactive FB material should be performed as soon as possible. The use of intravitreal and systemic antibiotics is controversial but usually performed to prevent endophthalmitis.

A 29-year-old man presents for a routine eye evaluation. His exam is normal except for the retinal exam.

1. What findings are depicted?
2. What is the differential diagnosis?
3. How would you work up this patient?

Additional information: the patient is HIV positive.

4. How would you treat him?

1. Multiple cotton wool spots (CWS), microaneurysms, and intraretinal hemorrhages.

2. The most common causes of CWS are diabetes and hypertension. Other causes include: ischemic (retinal vein occlusion, ocular ischemic syndrome, severe anemia, preeclampsia, carotid artery obstruction), embolic (carotid emboli, cardiac emboli, deep venous emboli, white blood cell emboli [Purtcher's retinopathy], severe chest compression/long bone fractures, foreign bodies [IVDA], amniotic fluid embolization), infectious (HIV, Rocky Mountain Spotted Fever, cat-scratch fever [*Bartonella henselae*], toxoplasmosis, subacute bacterial endocarditis, leptospirosis, onchocerciasis [river blindness], fungemia), toxic (interferon, methotrexate), radiation induced, neoplastic (lymphoma, leukemia, metastatic carcinoma, Hodgkin's disease), immune-mediated (systemic lupus erythematosis, sarcoidosis, dermatomyositis, polyarteritis nordosa, scleroderma, giant cell arteritis, cryoglobulinemia), traumatic nerve fiber layer laceration (note: CWS will not resolve), blood diseases (aplastic anemia, dysproteinemia, pernicious anemia [vitamin B12 deficiency]), hyperviscosity syndromes (multiple myeloma, Waldenström macroglobulinemia), hypercoagulability syndromes (factor V Leiden, prothrombin 20210A, hyperhomocysteinemia, protein S/C deficiency, antithrombin III deficiency, dysfibrinogenemia, factor XII deficiency), epiretinal membrane traction, and idiopathic.

3. A thorough history (radiation, chemotherapy, trauma) and review of systems are important to guide the laboratory evaluation. The patient needs a systemic workup for diabetes and hypertension. Initial blood tests include CBC and differential, platelet count, glycosylated hemoglobin, ANA, and HIV antibody test. Depending on the patient's cardiovascular risk factors, a workup looking for cardiac valvular disease, carotid stenosis or deep venous sources of emboli may be done. Infectious workup is based on other systemic symptoms.

4. No treatment is required for the retinopathy. The cotton wool spots resolve spontaneously within 1–2 months.

A 67-year-old woman noticed a sudden decrease in vision a few months ago.

1. What is the differential diagnosis?

2. How would you evaluate this patient?

Additional information: the OCT shows:

3. What is the diagnosis?

4. What are the risk factors?

5. What is the treatment?

6. What is the prognosis?

1. Macular hole, pseudohole, lamellar hole, cystoid macular edema, solar retinopathy (usually bilateral), epiretinal membrane, and exudative maculopathies including central serous chorioretinopathy (CSC) and wet age-related macular degeneration (AMD).

2. Perform a dilated fundus examination with evaluation for a Watzke–Allen sign (absolute scotoma in the hole).

    An optical coherence tomography (OCT) scan differentiates a macular hole from other entities including lamellar hole, pseudohole, solar retinopathy, cystoid macular edema, central serous chorioretinopathy, epiretinal membrane, and vitreomacular traction syndrome. It also illustrates intraretinal abnormalities including cystoid macular edema, intraretinal thickening, and the amount of traction on the edges of the hole. OCT is useful for staging the hole:

    Stage 1: premacular or impending hole with foveal detachment, decreased/absent foveal depression, and macular cyst (1A = yellow spot, 100–200 μm in diameter, 1B = yellow ring, 200–300 μm in diameter). There is no PVD, Weiss' ring, or vitreofoveal separation. Also known as vitreomacular traction since no full-thickness defect.
    Stage 2: early, small, full-thickness hole either centrally within the ring or eccentrically at the ring's margin. The OCT shows the partial thickness opening of the hole.
    Stage 3: full-thickness hole (<400 μm) often with yellow deposits at level of retinal pigment epithelium (Klein's tags), operculum over the hole within the hyaloid face, cuff of subretinal fluid at hole edges, cystoid macular edema at hole edges, absence of a Weiss ring, and positive Watzke–Allen sign (subjective interruption of slit beam on biomicroscopy).
    Stage 4: stage 3 and posterior vitreous detachment (PVD).

    A fluorescein angiogram (FA) is generally not required to differentiate this entity from others. It would show a window defect corresponding to the hole.

3. Stage 3 full-thickness macular hole with no vitreomaclar traction.

4. Cystoid macular edema, vitreomacular traction on the macula, trauma, postsurgical, postlaser treatment and postinflammatory disorders.

5. Stage 1 and many stage 2 holes are usually observed for spontaneous release of the hyaloid and hole closure. Stage 2 and higher holes are treated with pars plana vitrectomy with release of traction from the edges of the hole and placement of a nonexpansile, gas tamponade (usually sulfur hexafluoride) with face-down positioning for several days to 1 week after surgery. Vitreomacular traction (stage 1) and small full-thickness holes with traction (stage 2) are candidates for treatment with ocriplasmin (Jetrea), especially those <250 μ.

6. The prognosis depends on the duration and size of the hole. It is good for recent onset and smaller diameter holes, as well as patients with good preoperative visual acuity. The prognosis is poor for holes >1 year duration and >400 μm wide. Surgery is successful anatomically in 80–100% of cases depending on duration of the hole and hole width, with 65–85% of patients gaining three or more lines of visual acuity.

A 53-year-old man complains of photopsias and floaters for 2 days.

1. What finding does he have?

2. What is the diagnosis?

3. What other findings would you look for?

4. If the retinal exam is normal, how would you manage this patient?

Additional information: the patient returns in 1 month with an increase in symptoms and the following peripheral retinal appearance:

5. What is the diagnosis?

6. What are the risk factors?

7. What is the etiology?

8. What is the treatment?

1. Separation of the posterior hyaloid face from the retina with a Weiss ring.

2. Posterior vitreous detachment (PVD).

3. Retinal break (seen in 10–15% of acute, symptomatic PVDs) and rhegmatogenous retinal detachment (RD) especially when pigmented anterior vitreous cells are present, and vitreous hemorrhage (seen in 7.5% of acute, symptomatic PVDs) from a torn vessel during vitreous separation (70% risk of a retinal tear).

4. Instruct patient in the signs/symptoms of a retinal tear/detachment and repeat a dilated retinal exam in 4–6 weeks.

5. Retinal tear and rhegmatogenous retinal detachment.

6. Risk factors for retinal tears include age, history of RD in fellow eye (15%), high myopia/axial length (7%), family history, lattice degeneration, trauma, cataract surgery (1% after ICCE; 0.1% after ECCE with intact posterior capsule), diabetes, and Nd:YAG laser posterior capsulotomy.

7. Retinal tears occur when the vitreous detaches posteriorly and reaches a site with firmer attachment. The vitreous remains attached at the posterior margin of the retinal flap creating the horseshoe appearance. With additional traction, retinal tissue may avulse leading to an operculum over a round/oval hole.

8. Horseshoe tears and symptomatic retinal holes should be treated with laser photocoagulation or cryopexy to prevent retinal detachment. Asymptomatic retinal holes can be observed. In this case, the patient has developed a rhegmatogenous retinal detachment that requires surgical repair. If the tears are superior and localized to 1 clock hour, the patient is a candidate for pneumatic retinopexy. If not, a scleral buckle or primary pars plana vitrectomy should be performed.

A 57-year-old woman complains of blurred vision, nyctalopia, and peripheral photopsias in both eyes for 3 days.

1. What does the fundus photo show?

2. What is the differential diagnosis?

3. What ancillary studies would you obtain to make the diagnosis?

Additional information: laboratory testing reveals patient is positive for HLA-A29.

4. What is the diagnosis?

5. What other exam findings would you look for?

6. What is the epidemiology of this disease?

7. How would you treat this patient?

8. What is the prognosis?

1. Multiple, small, discrete, ovoid, creamy yellow-white spots at the level of the choroid and RPE scattered like a birdshot blast from a shotgun in the midperiphery radiating from the optic nerve. Notably, the lesions are not pigmented.

2. The differential diagnosis includes inflammatory disorders such as birdshot chorioretinopathy, other white dot syndromes (MEWDS, APMPPE), pars planitis, punctate inner choroidopathy, and sarcoidosis; infectious etiologies such as tuberculosis, syphilis, diffuse unilateral subacute neuroretinitis (DUSN), and toxoplasmosis; masquerade processes such as ocular lymphoma, metastatic disease, and choroidal lymphoproliferative diseases.

3. Laboratory testing for HLA typing would be most useful.

   An FA is useful to characterize the lesions. Birdshot lesions show mild hyperfluorescence early (active lesions may hypofluoresce early) and late staining. Late views show profuse vascular incompetence with leakage, petalloid cystoid macular edema, and secondary retinal staining. The phenomena of "quenching," where dye seems to disappear rapidly from the retinal circulation, can be seen in these patients.

4. Birdshot chorioretinopathy, also known as vitiliginous chorioretinitis, is associated with HLA-A29 (90–98%), although 7% of the general population is positive for HLA-A29.

5. Other signs of birdshot include mild vitritis, mild anterior chamber cells and flare (in 25% of cases), cystoid macular edema, retinal vasculitis, and variable amount of disc edema. Late findings include optic atrophy and epiretinal membranes. Macular CNV is rare.

6. Birdshot chorioretinopathy is a rare uveitis that occurs in 50- to 60-year-old females (70%) and almost exclusively in Caucasians of northern European descent.

7. Treatment is reserved for patients with decreased visual acuity, significant inflammation, or complications including cystoid macular edema.

   Despite historically poor responses to steroids, initial improvement can be seen with oral steroids. Intravitreal or subTenon's steroid injection is performed in patients with severe inflammation or cystoid macular edema. Early introduction of steroid-sparing agents, immunomodulatory agents including cyclosporine, azathioprine, mycophenolate mofetil, adalimumab, daclizumab, methotrexate, or intravenous polyclonal immunoglobulin can also be considered.

8. Birdshot is a chronic, slowly progressive, recurrent disease with variable visual prognosis. Most patients lose vision from chronic CME. Rarely, it is a selflimited disease.

A 28-year-old woman reports sudden vision loss in her left eye after having flu-like symptoms the week before.

1. What findings are shown?
2. What is the differential diagnosis?
3. How would you work up this patient?

Additional information: laboratory testing is positive for Bartonella henselae.

4. What is the diagnosis?
5. How would you treat this patient?
6. What is the prognosis?

1. Marked optic disc edema with disc hemorrhage and lipid exudation in a star shape.

2. The patient has a macular star exudate. Infectious etiologies to consider and rule out include *Bartonella henselae*, syphillis, Lyme disease, tuberculosis, tularemia, toxoplasmosis, viral retinitis (HSV, HZV, EBV), DUSN, and toxocariasis. Noninfectious etiologies to consider include hypertensive retinopathy, diabetic retinopathy, anterior ischemic optic neuropathy (AION), retinal vein occlusion, acute macular neuroretinopathy, sarcoidosis, and papilledema.

3. Check blood pressure. Laboratory testing for VDRL or RPR, FTA-ABS or MHA-TP, purified protein derivative (PPD), and indirect fluorescent antibody test for *Bartonella henselae*.

4. Neuroretinitis, also known as Leber's idiopathic stellate neuroretinitis, is due to a pleomorphic, Gram-negative, bacillus called *Bartonella henselae* (formerly known as *Rochalimaea*), which is associated with cat-scratch disease.

5. There are no definitive treatment guidelines given the selflimited and good prognosis. The use of systemic antibiotics (doxycycline, rifampin, tetracycline, ciprofloxacin, trimethoprim [Bactrim]) and steroids are controversial. The typical regimen for an immunocompetent patient is doxycycline for 2–4 weeks. For severe infections, intravenous doxycycline can be given along with rifampin.

6. Good with 67% regaining ≥20/20 vision, and 97% regaining >20/40 vision. The disc edema resolves over 8–12 weeks, whereas the macular star takes longer, resolving over 6–12 months. Optic atrophy and retinal pigment epithelial changes may develop late.

A 45-year-old man complains of blurred vision with metamorphopsia.

1. What does the photo depict?

2. What is the differential diagnosis?

3. What ancillary tests would you order?

4. What is the diagnosis?

5. What are the risk factors for this disease?

6. What other clinical findings are common?

Additional information: the FA shows:

7. How would you treat this patient?

8. What is the prognosis?

1. Small, round, yellow-brown, punched-out chorioretinal lesions (histo-spots) in the midperiphery and posterior pole, and juxtapapillary atrophic changes. In the macula there is a pigmented chorioretinal scar with choroidal neovascularization. The media is notably clear, indicating no vitreous haze.

2. In a patient of this age, choroidal neovascularization is usually due to presumed ocular histoplasmosis syndrome (POHS), pathologic myopia, or an inflammatory disorder such as multifocal choroiditis or punctate inner chorioretinopathy.

3. To verify that a CNV is present, an FA is most useful. An OCT or OCTA would also show the CNV. Laboratory testing is largely unnecessary, although histoplasmin antigen skin testing can be performed. It is important to note that 60% of the adult population of the Ohio and Mississippi River Valleys has a positive reaction to histoplasmin skin testing.

4. Presumed ocular histoplasmosis syndrome (POHS), caused by previous infection by the dimorphic fungus *Histoplasma capsulatum*, with secondary CNV.

5. Endemic in the Ohio and Mississippi river valleys, the fungus is present on feathers of chickens, pigeons, and blackbirds, in addition to infected bat droppings. Humans inhale fungus, which then disseminates into the bloodstream. POHS is rare in African Americans. It is associated with HLA-B7.

6. Over 60% of cases are bilateral. Most patients are asymptomatic unless they develop CNV. The four characteristic findings of POHS are: punched-out chorioretinal lesions (histo-spots), peripapillary atrophic pigmentary changes, lack of vitritis, and CNV:

   1. *Laser*: extra- and juxtafoveal CNV can be treated with focal laser photocoagulation. Subfoveal CNV should not be treated with laser (14% regress spontaneously).

   2. *Photodynamic therapy*: subfoveal CNV can be treated with ocular photodynamic therapy (PDT) with verteporfin (Visudyne).

   3. *Anti-VEGF*: although there are no randomized studies and no FDA-approved therapies for POHS, anti-VEGF agents (ranibizumab, bevacizumab, aflibercept, pegaptanib) are used to treat POHS related CNV with good success off-label.

   4. *Surgery*: removal of CNV with subretinal surgery was evaluated in Subretinal Surgery Trials (Group H); however, surgery was not found to be beneficial in patients with vision better than 20/100. Patients with vision worse than 20/100 had a better chance of improving vision over 2 years of follow-up. There was a high rate of CNV recurrence, cataract formation, and retinal detachment.

8. Better visual prognosis than CNV due to age-related macular degeneration with a 30% recurrence rate. Patients are at risk for CNV in the fellow eye (risk is less than 2% per year)

A 48-year-old woman has bilateral chronic vision loss.

1. What finding is present?
2. What is the differential diagnosis?
3. What tests would you obtain?
4. What other history would be helpful?

Additional information: the patient is being treated for systemic lupus erythematosis for 15 years.

5. What is the most likely diagnosis?
6. What are the risk factors for this problem?
7. How would you follow this patient?
8. How would you treat this patient?
9. What is the prognosis?

1. Retinal pigment epithelium depigmentation in a "bull's eye" configuration.

2. The differential diagnosis of a "bull's eye" maculopathy includes cone and cone–rod dystrophy, AMD, Stargardt disease/fundus flavimaculatus, central areolar choroidal dystrophy, benign concentric annular dystrophy, chloroquine/hydroxychloroquine retinal toxicity, chronic macular hole, olivopontocerebellar atrophy, and ceroid lipofuscinosis.

3. An FA would demonstrate the "bull's eye" pattern of hypofluorescence with a ring of hyperfluorescence that is often visible before the fundus lesion. It would rule out the "dark choroid" seen in Stargardt disease. Fundus autofluorescence would also demonstrate the bull's eye pattern. Humphrey visual field central 10–2 white-on-white pattern may demonstrate visual field defects. Multifocal ERG would show central depression. OCT shows thinning of the retina in the area of the bull's eye with absent inner/outer segment junction in a ring pattern (called flying saucer sign), which is very characteristic and obviates the need for FA in many patients. En-face OCT views are also helpful to see the bull's eye pattern.

4. It is important to ask the patient specifically about systemic lupus erythematosis, rheumatoid arthritis, short-term pulse treatment for graft versus host disease, and amebiasis, the use of toxic medications such as quinolones, and a history of any relatives with a similar eye problem to rule out a hereditary maculopathy.

5. Hydroxychloroquine retinal toxicity. Quinolones, first used as an antimalarial agent in World War II, are now used to treat systemic lupus erythematosis, rheumatoid arthritis, short-term pulse treatment for graft versus host disease, and amebiasis.

6. The major risk factors for retinal toxicity are daily dosage (most important; >5.0 mg/kg real weight for hydroxychloroquine, >2.3 mg/kg real weight for chloroquine), duration of use (>5 years with no other risk factors), renal disease, and concomitant tamoxifen use (5x increase risk). Other risk factors include liver disease, older age, and retinal/macular disease. The prevalence of toxicity is 7.5% among long-term users. The risk of developing hydroxychloroquine toxicity at recommended doses (<5.0 mg/kg/day) is <1% up to 5 years, <2% up to 10 years, but ~20% after 20 years.

7. The 2016 revised AAO recommendations on screening are as follows: a baseline ophthalmic exam within a year of starting the medication and visual field and spectral domain OCT if there is a maculopathy. Annual screenings beginning after 5 years of medication use or sooner if patient has major risk factors. High risk patients should be checked more frequently.

   Recommended screening tests: primary tests are automated visual fields (central 10 degrees (10-2) for non-Asians, paracentral scotoma; 24-2 or 30-2 for Asians, scotoma extends beyond macula) and/or SD OCT (ring of outer retinal thinning; flying saucer sign), and other objective tests are mfERG (enlarged a-wave, depressed b-wave) and fundus autofluorescence (reduced).

   Not recommended for screening are fundus examination, time domain OCT, FA, full-field ERG, Amsler grid, color testing, and EOG.

8. There is no treatment for hydroxychloroquine toxicity. Decrease or discontinue the medication to prevent central vision loss..

9. Retinopathy is not reversible and can even progress after the drug is discontinued.

A 19-year-old college student sees you for a new glasses prescription.

1. What does the photo reveal?
2. What is the differential diagnosis?
3. What other eye findings would you look for?

Additional information: slit-lamp examination with retroillumination shows:

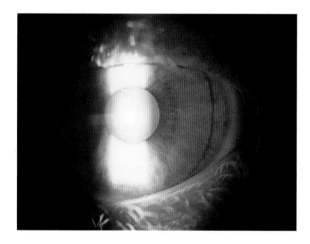

4. What is the diagnosis?
5. Describe the forms of this disease.
6. What are the risk factors for this disease?
7. How would you treat this patient?
8. What is the prognosis?

1. Generalized fundus hypopigmentation with the deep choroidal vasculature visible. There is foveal hypoplasia with no luteal pigment or foveal light reflex present.

2. Blond fundus (variant of normal) or ocular albinism.

3. Decreased vision, photophobia, high myopia, nystagmus, strabismus, pale irides with diffuse transillumination.

4. Ocular albinism.

5. Albinism is a congenital disorder of melanogenesis in which the synthesis of melanin is reduced or absent. Mutations in at least 13 genes can give rise to various forms of albinism depending on which structures are involved:

    Ocular albinism: this is a disorder, limited to the eye, with a decreased number of melanosomes (although each melanosome is fully pigmented).

    Oculocutaneous albinism: this is a systemic problem with decreased melanin in all melanosomes. These patients lack pigmentation of the hair, skin, and eyes. This form can further be categorized into tyrosinase positive (some pigmentation, which increases with age) and tyrosinase negative (no pigmentation). Two lethal variants of oculocutaneous albinism are:
    Chediak–Higashi: patients have reticuloendothelial incompetence with neutropenia, anemia, thrombocytopenia, recurrent infections, leukemia, and lymphoma.
    Hermansky–Pudlak: patients have clotting disorders and bleeding tendencies secondary to platelet abnormalities.

    All of the above forms of albinism can be further classified clinically based on the degree of ocular involvement:
    1. True albinism: patients have low visual acuity (20/100 to 20/400) and nystagmus due to hypoplasia of the fovea.
    2. Albinoidism: patients have normal or only slightly diminished visual acuity without nystagmus.

6. This is a heritable disease. Certain ethnic populations have a higher incidence. In particular, Africans and African Americans have a higher incidence than Caucasians, but often have incomplete forms of albinism.

7. There is no effective treatment. Refraction, tinted glasses, and low vision aids are helpful for older patients. Medical and hematology consultation is advisable to rule out potentially lethal variants. All forms of albinism are heritable, necessitating genetic counseling.

8. The prognosis is variable depending on the form of albinism. This disease is not degenerative, however, and visual acuity can even improve over the first two decades of life.

A 36-year-old man presents with decreased vision in his left eye.

1. What are the retinal findings?
2. What is the most likely diagnosis and what tests can be performed to confirm it?
3. What is the differential diagnosis?
4. What additional ophthalmic tests would be helpful?

1. Numerous intraretinal hemorrhages, microaneurysms, cotton-wool spots, and lipid exudates scattered throughout the posterior pole. No retinal or optic nerve neovascularization, preretinal hemorrhage, or vitreous hemorrhage is seen.

2. Diabetic retinopathy. Check serum hemoglobin A1c, fasting blood sugar, and blood pressure.

3. Hypertensive retinopathy, retinopathies associated with blood disorders, radiation retinopathy, retinal vein occlusion, ocular ischemic syndrome, parafoveal telangiectasia, and Eales' disease.

4. A fluorescein angiogram (FA) would be useful to evaluate macular ischemia and to rule out neovascularization. An optical coherence tomography (OCT) scan would be useful to evaluate for the presence of posterior hyaloidal traction, epiretinal proliferation, and the nature of the macular edema (diffuse vs focal). OCT angiography (OCTA) can show retinal ischemia and microaneurysms.

5. What level of retinopathy does this patient exhibit?

6. How would you manage this patient?

7. This patient has proliferative diabetic retinopathy in his fellow eye. How would you treat it?

5. Diabetic retinopathy can be classified based on the clinical features. This patient has very severe nonproliferative diabetic retinopathy defined by the "4-2-1 rule": (4) intraretinal hemorrhages and/or microaneurysms in all 4 quadrants; or (2) venous beading in at least 2 quadrants; or (1) intraretinal microvascular abnormality (IRMA) in at least 1 quadrant. Very severe NPDR exists if there is more than one of these features, as in this case.

6. 1. Medical: the Diabetes Control and Complications Trial (DCCT) and United Kingdom Prospective Diabetes Study (UKPDS) concluded that tight blood sugar and blood pressure control slowed progression of retinopathy, development of macular edema, need for treatment, and other microvascular complications.

   2. Anti-VEGF: for macular edema involving the fovea (center-involving), ranibizumab (Lucentis; DRCR.net Protocol I, DRCR.net Protocol T, RISE, RIDE, RESTORE, and RESOLVE studies), aflibercept (Eylea; DRCR.net Protocol T, VIVID, VISTA studies) and bevacizumab (Avastin; DRCR.net Protocol T) have been shown to be very effective therapies. This patient would be an ideal candidate for intravitreal anti-VEGF therapy. Protocol T suggests that if the vision was worse than 20/50 then aflibercept may be the best choice, but if the vision was better, then any of the three anti-VEGF agents would work. In year 2 of Protocol T, there was no difference between aflibercept and ranibizumab, but bevacizumab was not as effective.

   3. Laser: the Early Treatment Diabetic Retinopathy Study (EDTRS) concluded that focal/grid laser photocoagulation decreased moderate visual loss by 50% in patients with clinically significant macular edema (CSME) defined as: (1) retinal thickening within 500 µm of the macular center *or* (2) hard exudates within 500 µm of the macular center with adjacent thickening *or* (3) zone of retinal thickening 1 disc area in size any portion of which is within 1 disc diameter of the macular center. CSME is based only on clinical examination and not visual acuity (treat even with 20/20 vision) or other imaging studies. Laser treatment is second line to anti-VEGF therapy.

   4. Steroids: considered third-line therapy behind laser and anti-VEGF therapy, intraocular steroids have been shown to be effective especially in patients who are already pseudophakic. Although the Diabetic Retinopathy Clinical Trials Network (DRCR.net) Protocol B did not find steroids better than laser in the overall study population, DRCR.net Protocol I did show a benefit in pseudophakic patients. Similarly, the sustained release, fluocinolone acetonide, steroid implant (Iluvien) has been shown to be effective over a 3-year follow-up period in patients who had previous laser therapy and persistent edema (FAME Study). Finally, the dexamthesone implant (Ozuredex) has been found to be effective (MEAD Study). With all steroids, careful monitoring of cataract formation and IOP is important.

   5. Surgery: if a patient exhibits posterior hyaloidal traction then pars plana vitrectomy with membrane peel should be considered. This patient did not exhibit any traction.

7. The first question would be to decide if the patient had high-risk characteristics or not. The Diabetic Retinopathy Study (DRS) concluded that, in the presence of high-risk characteristics, immediate panretinal photocoagulation (PRP) should be instituted.

   High-risk characteristics of PDR are defined as: neovascularization of the disc (NVD) > standard photo 10A used in DRS (one-third to one-quarter disc area) *or* any NVD and VH or preretinal hemorrhage *or* neovascularization elsewhere (NVE) > standard photo 7 (one-half disc area) and VH or preretinal hemorrhage.

A 26-year-old man says he has noted trouble with night driving.

1. What does the picture show?
2. What is the differential diagnosis?

Additional examination: an electroretinogram (ERG) shows markedly reduced/absent a-wave and b-wave amplitudes and implicit times.

3. What is the diagnosis?
4. What other eye findings are associated with this disease?

1. Dark pigmentary clumps in the midperiphery and perivenous areas (bone spicules), attenuated retinal vessels, and waxy optic disc pallor.

2. Bone spicules and disc pallor are found in retinitis pigmentosa, congenital rubella syndrome, syphilis, thioridazine/chloroquine drug toxicity, carcinoma-associated retinopathy, congenital stationary night blindness, vitamin A deficiency, trauma, and diffuse unilateral subacute neuroretinitis.

3. Retinitis pigmentosa (RP).

4. Posterior subcapsular cataracts, high myopia, astigmatism, keratoconus, constricted visual fields, dyschromatopsia, and mild hearing loss (30%, excluding Usher's patients). Fifty percent of female carriers with the X-linked form have a golden reflex in the posterior pole.

5. Describe the various forms of this disease and their classification.

5. There are more than 29 loci associated with various phenotypes of RP with more being discovered daily.

Atypical forms:

Retinitis pigmentosa inversus: the macula and posterior pole are primarily affected so this form is confused with hereditary macular disorders. Central and color vision are reduced earlier than normal and pericentral ring/central scotomas occur.

Retinitis pigmentosa sine pigmento: this is a descriptive term for patients with symptoms of retinitis pigmentosa, but who fail to show pigmentary fundus changes. It is seen in up to 20% of cases and is associated with more pronounced cone dysfunction.

Retinitis punctata albescens (autosomal recessive [AR]): multiple, punctate white (50–100 μm) spots at the level of the retinal pigment epithelium are scattered in the midperiphery with attenuated vessels and bone spicules. This is a slowly progressive disease, which differentiates it from fundus albipunctatus.

Sector retinitis pigmentosa: this form has pigmentary changes limited to one retinal area that generally does not enlarge, usually in the inferonasal quadrants, and therefore the ERG responses are relatively good.

Forms associated with systemic abnormalities:

Abetalipoproteinemia (Bassen-Kornzweig syndrome)(AR): this form has minimal pigmentary changes early and is associated with ataxia, steatorrhea, erythrocyte acanthocytosis, growth retardation, neuropathy, and lack of serum beta-lipoprotein causing intestinal malabsorption of fat-soluble vitamins (A, D, E, K), triglycerides, and cholesterol.

Alstrom's disease (AR): this form has early profound visual loss and is associated with cataracts, deafness, obesity, renal failure, acanthosis nigricans, baldness, and hypogenitalism.

Cockayne's syndrome: this form is associated with band keratopathy, cataracts, dwarfism, deafness, intracranial calcifications, and psychosis.

Kearns–Sayre syndrome (AR): this form is associated with chronic, progressive external ophthalmoplegia, ptosis, cardiac conduction defects (arrhythmias, heart block, cardiomyopathy), and other abnormalities. "Ragged red" fibers are seen histologically on muscle biopsy.

Laurence–Moon/Bardet–Biedl syndromes (AR): Bardet–Biedl (polydactyly in 75% and syndactyly in 14%) and Laurence–Moon (spastic paraplegia, no polydactyly/syndactyly). Both forms have minimal pigmentary changes early and are characterized by short stature, congenital obesity, hypogenitalism (50%), partial deafness (5%), renal abnormalities, and mental retardation (85%).

Neuronal ceroid lipofuscinosis (Batten disease) (AR): this form can have infantile (Hagberg–Santavuori syndrome), juvenile, or adult onset and is associated with seizures, dementia, ataxia, and mental retardation. Conjunctival biopsy shows granular inclusions with autofluorescent lipopigments that also accumulate in neurons causing the retinal and CNS degeneration.

Refsum's disease (AR): this form has minimal pigmentary changes early and is associated with ichthyosis, EKG abnormalities, anosmia, deafness, progressive peripheral neuropathy, cerebellar ataxia, hypotonia, hepatomegaly, mental retardation, and elevated CSF protein. It is caused by a defect in fatty acid metabolism due to phytanic acid oxidase deficiency. This results in elevated plasma phytanic acid, pipecolic acid, and very long-chain fatty acid levels.

Usher's syndrome (AR): this form is associated with congenital, neurosensory hearing loss. It is the most common syndrome associated with retinitis pigmentosa (5%), and there are four types: type I (total deafness with no vestibular function), type II (partial deafness with normal vestibular function, most common type (67%), better vision), type III (Hallgren's syndrome = deafness, vestibular ataxia, psychosis), type IV (deafness and mental retardation).

6. How would you treat this patient?

7. What is the prognosis?

6. For most forms including this patient there is no effective treatment, but some patients respond to oral vitamin A therapy that slows reduction of ERG amplitudes and avoidance of vitamin E. When patients are placed on this therapy, liver function tests and serum retinol levels should be checked annually. In addition, treatment should include obtaining the best visual potential for the patient including correcting any refractive error, prescribing dark glasses, and low vision consultation for visual aids.

7. The prognosis is usually poor. Most patients are legally blind by the 4th decade of life.

A 70-year-old man presents with blurred vision in his left eye. He notes having intermittent photopsias over the past 3 months in that eye, but became concerned when he developed a visual field defect.

1. What does the photo reveal?

2. What etiology do you suspect?

3. What other tests would you order?

Additional information: a fine needle biopsy is obtained.

4. What does the pathology show?

5. What is the recommended treatment?

6. How would you follow this patient after treatment?

7. What is the prognosis?

8. What are the complications of radiation therapy?

1. A brown, domed-shaped mass with overlying exudative retinal detachment.

2. Choroidal malignant melanoma.

3. The most important test is ultrasound to differentiate between a tumor and other diseases in the differential diagnosis. The B-scan would show the tumor and the shape of the tumor (eg, mushroom, dome, or biconvex shape). The A-scan in a choroidal malignant melanoma would show low to medium internal reflectivity with reduction in amplitude from front to back, and high-amplitude spikes consistent with break in Bruch's membrane. Careful examination must be performed to evaluate for extrascleral extension. A fluorescein angiogram (FA) would show "double" circulation within the tumor from filling of both the retinal and choroidal vasculature. The lesion itself would be hypofluorescent early with pinpoint leakage late. Although not required, neuroimaging can be performed (a melanoma is bright on T1 and dark on T2 MRI imaging).

4. This specimen demonstrates epithelioid cells. Histopathology is based on the Callender classification:

   Spindle A cells are slender with cigar-shaped nucleus and finely dispersed chromatin. They have a low nuclear-to-cytoplasmic ratio, absent or inconspicuous nucleolus, and no mitotic figures. These tumors carry the best prognosis (5-year survival rate = 95%).
   Spindle B cells are oval with larger nucleus containing mitotic figures and coarser chromatin and prominent nucleolus. Epithelioid cells are polyhedral with abundant cytoplasm and a large, round-to-oval nucleus with peripheral margination of chromatin and prominent eosinophilic or purple nucleolus. The cells are poorly cohesive with distinct borders. Epithelioid cells are the most malignant and carry the worst prognosis (5-year survival <30%).

5. Treatment is based on the size of the tumor defined in the Collaborative Ocular Melanoma Study (COMS):

   1. Small tumors (apical height = 1.5–2.4 mm and basal diameter = 5–16 mm): there is no clear treatment choice, so these tumors can be observed closely if they are very small. Risk factors for growth of small melanomas are based on the following findings: thickness >2 mm, subretinal fluid, symptoms, orange pigment, margin <3 mm from optic disc, ultrasound hollow, halo absent, drusen absent (0 factors risk = 4%, each risk increases relative risk approximately 3×).

   2. Medium tumors (apical height = 2.5–10 mm and basal diameter ≤16 mm): since survival rates were similar between enucleation and iodine-125 plaque brachytherapy, the treatment of choice is radiation with either a high-energy radiation source (cobalt-60, iridium-192), low-energy radiation source (iodine-125, palladium-106, ruthenium-106), or charged particle radiation (proton beam).

   3. Large tumors (apical height >10 mm and basal diameter >16 mm; without metastasis. Updated definition is apical height >2 mm and basal diameter >16 mm, or apical height >10 mm regardless of basal diameter, or apical height >8 mm and <2 mm from optic disc): since preenucleation radiation did not change the survival rate in patients with large choroidal melanomas with or without metastases over enucleation alone, the treatment of choice is enucleation.

   This patient should be treated with enucleation.

6. Patients need to be observed closely for metastasis. The most common sites of metastasis are the liver, lung, bone, skin, and central nervous system; therefore annual liver function tests and chest imaging should be performed.

7. Approximately 50% of patients with large tumors have metastasis within 5 years with a mean survival after metastasis of 9 months.

8. The main complications are radiation retinopathy, cataracts (posterior subcapsular in 42% within 3 years of proton beam therapy), and dry eye. There is a high risk of substantial visual loss from I–125 brachytherapy (up to 49%) and patients must understand that the therapy is to treat the tumor and not vision.

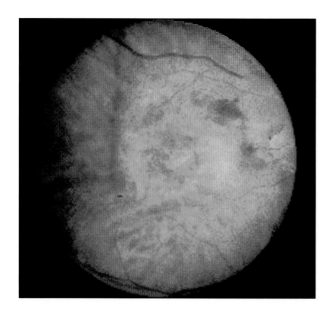

An 85-year-old woman presents with new distortion of vision in her right eye.

1. What does the photo show?

2. What is the differential diagnosis?

3. What tests would you perform?

Additional information: the FA shows:

4. What is the most likely diagnosis?

5. What treatment would you recommend?

6. How would you follow this patient?

1. Subretinal fluid and hemorrhage.

2. In a patient this age, the differential diagnosis includes exudative age-related macular degeneration (AMD), atypical central serous chorioretinopathy (CSC), adult vitelliform lesion, and other causes of choroidal neovascularization (CNV) including presumed ocular histoplasmosis (POHS), inflammatory, pathologic myopia, and idiopathic.

3. The key test is a fluorescein angiogram (FA) to verify the presence of a choroidal neovascular membrane and rule out other causes of fluid and hemorrhage. Indocyanine green (ICG) angiography would be useful to evaluate for central serous chorioretinopathy and polypoidal choroidal vasculopathy (PCV). Finally, optical coherence tomography (OCT) would verify the presence of fluid, CNV, and rule out other causes such as a thickened choroid with central serous chorioretinopathy, or a vitelliform lesion, and OCT angiography (OCTA) would show CNV.

4. Exudative age-related macular degeneration.

5. Since the CNV is subfoveal, the patient is not a candidate for laser photocoagulation:

   1. *Anti-VEGF*: for CNV involving the fovea, ranibizumab (Lucentis; MARINA, ANCHOR, CATT, IVAN, MANTA, GEFAL studies), bevacizumab (Avastin; CATT, IVAN, MANTA, GEFAL studies), and aflibercept (Eylea; VIEW studies) have been shown to be equally effective therapies when given monthly, while aflibercept was also shown to be equally effective to monthly ranibizumab when given every 8 weeks. Pegaptanib (Macugen) does not have similar visual results and is not first line therapy. This patient would be a candidate for anti-VEGF therapy.

   2. *Ocular photodynamic therapy with verteporfin (Visudyne)*: can be used alone (TAP, VIP studies) or in combination with anti-VEGF agents (DENALI, MT BLANC studies) with results of combination therapy similar to anti-VEGF alone. In general, PDT is a second-line therapy unless patient has polypoidal choroidal vasculopathy, where it may offer benefits over anti-VEGF alone.

6. The CATT Study reported that as-needed therapy gives similar results to monthly therapy but required monthly monitoring. Thus, monthly monitoring with clinical examination and OCT evaluation should be performed to evaluate for evidence of CNV activity. Retreatment should be performed when there is evidence of disease activity.

Additional information: the appearance of the patient's fellow eye is shown.

7. What would you recommend for this eye?

8. The patient's 62-year-old son has extensive intermediate drusen in both maculas. What treatment recommendations would you give him?

9. What is the son's prognosis?

7. There is no therapy for geographic atrophy so the patient should be counseled about low-vision aids.

8. The Age-related Eye Disease Study (AREDS) reported that supplements with high-dose antioxidants and zinc (vitamin C, 500 mg; vitamin E, 400 IU; and beta carotene, 15 mg, zinc, 80 mg and copper, 2 mg) are helpful in reducing vision loss and the progression of disease in patients with category 3 and 4 AMD. The AREDS classification is:

   Category 1: fewer than 5 small (<63 μm) drusen.
   Category 2 (mild AMD): multiple small drusen or single or nonextensive intermediate (63–124 μm) drusen, or pigment abnormalities.
   Category 3 (intermediate AMD): extensive intermediate-sized drusen, or 1 or more large (>125 μm) drusen, or noncentral geographic atrophy.
   Category 4 (advanced AMD): vision loss (<20/32) due to AMD in 1 eye (due to either central/subfoveal geographic atrophy or exudative macular degeneration).

   The AREDS2 Study, which evaluated lutein, zeaxanthin, and omega-3 fatty acids in addition to the original AREDS formulation, found that current smokers should avoid high-dose beta carotene (increased risk of lung cancer), adding lutein and zeaxanthin is beneficial (~20% reduction in disease progression beyond original AREDS in patients who had the lowest dietary intake of lutein and zeaxanthin), and there was no additional benefit from omega-3 fatty acids. As a result, the AREDS formula was adjusted by removing betacarotene and adding lutein and zeaxanthin.

   Thus, the patient's son should be placed on the AREDS2 supplementation and counseled to monitor his central vision for changes with an Amsler grid.

9. The rate of progression to advanced AMD over 5 years was 1.3% in eyes with many small or few medium drusen (if both eyes have many intermediate drusen, but no large drusen, then patient score = 1 in scale below), and 18% in eyes with many medium or any large drusen (as in this patient).

   Another method to calculate risk is the AREDS Clinical Severity Scale that is based on giving one point for the presence of ≥1 large drusen and/or pigment changes (either hyper, hypo, or noncentral GA) per eye, or 2 points for advanced AMD in one eye, then total the points for the two eyes to obtain a point score that shows the risk of developing advanced AMD in 5 years:

   0 points = 0.5%
   1 point = 3%
   2 points = 12%
   3 points = 25%
   4 points = 50%

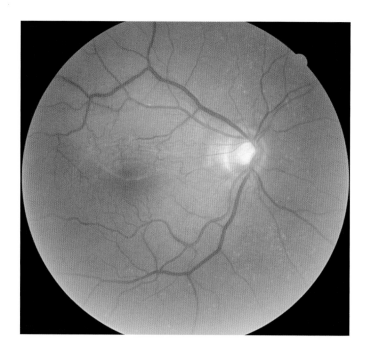

A 63-year-old woman is frustrated because of increasing difficulty reading the newspaper over the past 6 months.

1. What retinal findings are shown?

2. What symptoms may occur?

3. How would you evaluate this patient?

1. There is a thin, translucent membrane with dragged/tortuous vessels and retinal striae especially evident in the superior macula.

2. Metamorphopsia, macropsia, and decreased vision.

3. Visual acuity and Amsler grid testing is useful for monitoring the effect on visual function.

   An OCT scan demonstrates the amount of traction produced and differentiates this from other entities including epiretinal membrane, lamellar hole, pseudohole, macular hole, and vitreomacular traction syndrome. It also illustrates intraretinal abnormalities including cystoid macular edema, intraretinal thickening, and subretinal fluid.

   An FA shows the degree of retinal vascular tortuosity, retinal vascular leakage, and macular edema. The presence of macular edema may indicate a worse visual prognosis.

Additional information: her OCT shows:

4. What is the diagnosis?

5. What are the risk factors?

6. What is the treatment?

7. What are the complications of surgery?

8. What is the prognosis after surgery?

4. Epiretinal membrane (ERM) with cystoid macular edema.

5. Although most epiretinal membranes are idiopathic and occur in women older than 50 years of age, risk factors include prior intraocular surgery, intraocular inflammation, retinal vascular occlusion, sickle cell retinopathy, telangiectasia, diabetic retinopathy, arteriole macroaneurysm, previous vitreous hemorrhage, trauma, macular holes, intraocular tumors such as angiomas and hamartomas, telangiectasis, retinal arteriolar macroaneurysms, inherited retinal dystrophies such as retinitis pigmentosa, previous laser photocoagulation, and previous cryotherapy.

6. An ERM rarely requires treatment. Pars plana vitrectomy and membrane peel are considered in patients with reduced acuity (<20/40) or who are symptomatic.

7. The most common complication is cataracts (nuclear sclerosis; posterior subcapsular is due to lens touch or the use of intraocular gas). Retinal tears occur in up to 5% of cases. The most common late complication is rhegmatogenous retinal detachment (probably as a result of contraction of the vitreous into the sclerotomy sites). Rare complications include phototoxicity (especially when intraocular dyes such as ICG are used), endophthalmitis, and visual field defects.

8. 80–90% of patients have an improvement in visual acuity of 2 or more Snellen lines. Recurrent ERM occurs in up to 5% of patients.

5/23/2011
2

A 65-year-old man presents with a sudden, painless, quadrantic visual field defect.

1. What does the fundus photo show?
2. What is the differential diagnosis?
3. What test would you obtain?

1. Dilated, tortuous, superior retinal vein with superficial, retinal hemorrhages, and cotton-wool spots in a wedge-shaped area radiating from an arteriovenous crossing.

2. Branch retinal vein occlusion, venous stasis retinopathy, ocular ischemic syndrome, hypertensive retinopathy, leukemic retinopathy, retinopathy of anemia, diabetic retinopathy, papilledema, papillophlebitis (in young patients).

3. Fluorescein angiography (FA); consider a wide-field FA to evaluate for peripheral ischemia. OCT is often also performed to evaluate for amount and location of macular edema. OCTA shows the ischemic areas and can delineate neovascularization.

Additional information: the FA shows:

4. How do you interpret this test?

5. What is the diagnosis?

6. What are the risk factors for this disease?

7. What are the different forms?

8. How would you work up this patient?

9. What is the treatment?

10. What is the prognosis?

4. The FA shows delayed retinal venous filling in the superior branch of the central retinal vein, blocked fluorescence from retinal hemorrhages, and capillary nonperfusion in the area supplied by the involved retinal vein.

5. Branch retinal vein occlusion

6. Retinal vein occlusion (RVO) is associated with hypertension (50–70% of cases), coronary artery disease, diabetes mellitus, and peripheral vascular disease. Rare associations include: hypercoagulable states (eg, macroglobulinemia, cryoglobulinemia), hyperviscosity states (polycythemia vera, Waldenström's macroglobulinemia), systemic lupus erythematosus, syphilis, sarcoid, homocystinuria, malignancies (eg, multiple myeloma, polycythemia vera, leukemia), optic nerve drusen, and external compression. In younger patients, associated with oral contraceptive pills, collagen vascular disease, acquired immunodeficiency syndrome (AIDS), protein S/protein C/antithrombin III deficiency, factor XII (Hageman factor) deficiency, antiphospholipid antibody syndrome, or activated protein C resistance (factor V Leiden polymerase chain reaction [PCR] assay).

7. There are two types of RVO: nonischemic (64%) and ischemic (defined as ≥ 5 disc areas of capillary nonperfusion on FA).

8. In older patients, obtain fasting blood glucose, glycosylated hemoglobin and blood pressure measurement to rule out hypertension and diabetes. Consider checking: CBC with differential, platelets, PT/PTT, antinuclear antibody (ANA), rheumatoid factor (RF), angiotensin converting enzyme (ACE), ESR, serum protein electrophoresis, lipid profile, hemoglobin electrophoresis (in African American), sedimentation rate, Venereal Disease Research Laboratory (VDRL) or Rapid Plasma Reagin (RPR), treponemal antibody absorption test (FTA-ABS) or microhemagglutination for treponema pallidum (MHA-TP) depending on the clinical situation.

   In younger patients ($<$40 years old) and in whom a hypercoagulable state is being considered, check: human immunodeficiency virus (HIV) status, functional protein S assay, functional protein C assay, functional antithrombin III assay (type II heparin-binding mutation), antiphospholipid antibody titer, lupus anticoagulant, anticardiolipin antibody titer (IgG and IgM), homocysteine level (if elevated test for folate, B12, and creatinine), factor XII (Hageman factor) levels, and activated protein C resistance (factor V Leiden mutation PCR assay). If these tests are normal and clinical suspicion for a hypercoagulable state still exists, then order: plasminogen antigen assay, heparin cofactor II assay, thrombin time, reptilase time, and fibrinogen functional assay.

9. 1. <u>Anti-VEGF:</u> the BRAVO Study reported better results than laser using monthly intravitreal injection of ranibizumab (Lucentis) for macular edema. Bevacizumab is used off-label for macular edema. The VIBRANT Study reported better results than laser using monthly intravitreal injection of aflibercept (Eylea) for six injections, then every other month. Anti-VEGF is the first-line therapy. If vision is good, the practitioner can observe to see if spontaneous resolution occurs.

   2. <u>Laser:</u> the BVOS reported that macular grid/focal photocoagulation should be performed when macular edema lasts $>$3 months and vision is worse than 20/40. If rubeosis, disc/retinal neovascularization, or neovascular glaucoma develops, then quadrantic scatter laser photocoagulation to the area of ischemia. Prophylactic laser was not evaluated in the BVOS and is not recommended.

   3. <u>Steroids:</u> the GENEVA (Global Evaluation of Implantable Dexamethasone in Retinal Vein Occlusion with Macular Edema) Study reported positive results using an intravitreal injection of a sustained release intravitreal dexamethasone implant (Ozurdex) for macular edema.

10. Thirty percent have spontaneous recovery and $>$50% maintain vision better than 20/40 after 1 year. Ten percent have BRVO in the fellow eye.

A 22-year-old woman reports decreased vision with photopsias.

1. What does the fundus photo show?

2. What is the differential diagnosis?

3. What test would you obtain?

Additional information: the FA shows:

4. How do you interpret this test?

5. What is the diagnosis?

6. What are the risk factors for this disease?

7. What is the treatment?

8. What is the prognosis?

1. Multifocal, deep gray-white retinal lesions with orange yellow granularity of the fovea.

2. White dot syndrome including multiple evanescent white dot syndrome (MEWDS), acute posterior multifocal placoid pigment epitheliopathy (APMPPE), mulifocal choroiditis and panuveitis (MCP), punctate inner choroiditis (PIC), and birdshot chorioretinopathy.

3. Fluorescein angiography (FA; see below), fundus autofluorescence (FAF) shows hyper-autofluorescent areas corresponding to lesions. OCT shows discontinuities in the outer retina (outer segment ellipsoid zone and ELM) corresponding to the lesions. Enlarged blind spot and central or paracentral scotoma on visual field testing. ICG show hyperfluorescent lesions that outnumber fundus lesions.

4. The FA demonstrates early punctate hyperfluorescence in a wreath-like pattern with late staining that correspond to the lesions.

5. MEWDS.

6. Healthy young woman aged 15–50 years old; may be associated with prodromal viral illness.

7. No treatment needed; selflimited disease.

8. Good, but up to 10% can have recurrences.

A 75-year-old woman presents with sudden, painless, loss of vision.

1. What does the fundus photo show?

2. What is the differential diagnosis?

3. What testing may be helpful?

Additional information: if the FA shows:

4. What is the diagnosis?

5. What are the risk factors for this disease?

6. How would you work up this patient?

7. What is the treatment?

8. What is the prognosis?

1. Cherry red spot.

2. The differential diagnosis of a cherry red spot is mainly central retinal artery occlusion and metabolic storage diseases such as Hurler's disease, Tay–Sachs disease (GM2 gangliosidosis), MPS VII (Sly syndrome), Farber's disease, GM1 gangliosidoses, Niemann Pick's disease, Sandhoff disease, Shprintzen–Goldberg syndrome, Hallervorden Spatz disease, Krabbe disease, metachromatic leukodystrophy; also trauma (commotio retinae), ophthalmic artery occlusion (cherry red spot may be present but usually is not), and toxicity from methanol, quinine, dapsone, and carbon monoxide,

3. FA shows delayed filling of retinal arteries and delayed arteriovenous transit time. OCT in acute shows increased reflectivity and thickening of the inner retina, and decreased reflectivity of the outer retina. Late OCT shows retina thinning. OCTA shows the areas of non-perfusion.

4. Central retinal artery occlusion with patent cilioretinal artery.

5. Atherosclerosis, cardiac valvular disease, hypercoagulable states including oral contraceptive use, and collagen vascular diseases.

6. Carotid Doppler ultrasound and cardiac echocardiography. In older patients, obtain ESR and C-reactive protein to rule out giant cell arteritis. If work up is negative, then consider laboratory tests for hypercoagulable state depending on the clinical situation.

7. There is no effective treatment. Any chance of success to limit visual loss must be instituted within 90 minutes of onset making intervention unlikely. All attempts at treatment are based on the idea of moving the embolus (ie, lowering IOP rapidly with anterior chamber paracentesis, systemic acetazolamide, digital ocular massage, topical ocular hypotensive drops, carbogen treatment), and should be performed before imaging tests to prevent vision loss.

8. Poor prognosis. In the presence of cilioretinal artery sparing CRAO, visual prognosis is better with 80% having 20/50 or better vision. Neovascular complications can occur in 15–20% of patients.

A 62-year-old woman complains of gradual decreased vision OD. Her BSCVA is 20/50 with a mild hyperopic shift.

1. What does the fundus photo show?

2. What is the diagnosis and differential diagnosis?

3. What are the possible etiologies?

4. What tests would you obtain?

Additional information: The patient underwent uncomplicated cataract surgery 3 months ago. The FA shows:

5. What does the FA demonstrate?

6. What is the diagnosis?

7. What are the risk factors for this disease?

8. What is the treatment?

1. Decreased foveal reflex with intraretinal cystic changes.

2. Cystoid macular edema CME). The differential diagnosis of CME is pseudocystoid macular edema (no leakage on FA; x-linked retinoschisis, Goldmann–Favre syndrome, and nicotinic acid maculopathy), macular hole (stage 1), macular pseudohole, foveal retinoschisis, central serous chorioretinopathy, choroidal neovascular membrane.

3. The etiology of CME can be remembered with the mnemonic: DEPRIVEN (**D**iabetes, **E**pinephrine, **P**ars planitis, **R**P, **I**rvine-Gass syndrome, **V**enous occlusion, **E**$_2$ prostaglandin, **N**icotinic acid maculopathy (does not leak). However, this is not a complete list, and other causes include uveitis, macular or retinal telangiectasia, retinal vasculitis, epiretinal membrane, hereditary retinal dystrophies (dominant CME as well as RP), hypertensive retinopathy, radiation retinopathy, exudative AMD, occult rhegmatogenous RD, intraocular tumors, collagen vascular diseases, hypotony, and chronic inflammation.

4. Fluorescein angiography (FA; see below), OCT shows the typical cystoid spaces with loss of the normal foveal contour and increased retinal thickening; may also show subretinal fluid.

5. Leakage from perifoveal capillaries with petalloid appearance.

6. Pseudophakic cystoid macular edema (Irvine–Gass syndrome).

7. Clinical CME is rare after uncomplicated small incision phacoemulsification cataract extraction occurring in 2–5% of cases; however, angiographic or OCT based CME is seen in 15–30% of cases. In complicated cases, reports as high as 60%. Risk factors include diabetic retinopathy, uveitis, glaucoma (especially with prostaglandin analog therapy), retinal vein occlusion, and preexisting epiretinal membrane.

8. Topical NSAID drops are usually tried first (a meta-analysis of four randomized clinical trials showed a benefit). A combination of steroid and NSAID drops are added in more resistant cases. Periocular and intravitreal steroids, and anti-VEGF injections have been used in difficult cases.

A 72-year-old woman is found to have a fundus abnormality on routine examination.

1. What does the fundus photo show?

2. What is the differential diagnosis?

3. What test would you obtain?

Additional information: the FA shows:

4. What is the diagnosis?

5. What are the risk factor(s) for this disease?

6. What is the treatment?

1. Lipid exudates and hemorrhage surrounding a focal dilation of a retinal artery.

2. Retinal artery macroaneurysm, Coats' disease, von Hippel–Lindau, branch retinal vein occlusion, diabetic retinopathy, radiation retinopathy.

3. Fluorescein angiogram (FA), if too much blood then ICG angiogram should be performed.

4. Retinal artery macroaneurysm.

5. Strong association with hypertension.

6. Usually none required; often spontaneously regress after bleed. Anti-VEGF agents have been tried with success when macular edema occurs in association with the macroaneurysm. In the past, laser treatment adjacent to the macroaneurysm has been reported, but is controversial. In severe bleeding, surgery has been advocated especially with submacular hemorrhage or nonclearing vitreous hemorrhage.

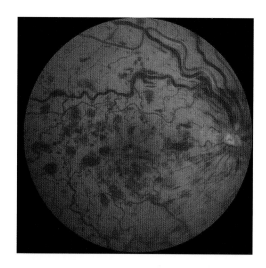

A 73-year-old man presents with painless, sudden decrease in vision that he noticed upon awakening.

1. What does the fundus photo show?
2. What is the differential diagnosis?
3. What testing would you obtain?

Additional information: the FA shows:

4. What does the FA show, and what is the diagnosis?
5. What are the risk factors for this disease?
6. What are the different forms?
7. What laboratory evaluation should be performed?
8. What is the treatment?
9. What is the prognosis?

1. Disc edema with tortuous, dilated retinal veins and intraretinal hemorrhages in all 4 quadrants.

2. Central retinal vein occlusion, hemiretinal vein occlusion, branch retinal vein occlusion, ocular ischemic syndrome, radiation retinopathy, retinal artery occlusion, acute retinal necrosis.

3. FA to evaluate arteriovenous transit time and nonperfusion; wide angle FA is helpful to evaluate the extent of non-perfusion. OCT to evaluate for macular edema.

4. The FA shows no filling of the central retinal vein and blocking from hemorrhages, which is characteristic of a central retinal vein occlusion.

5. Risk factors for a CRVO include age (90% of cases >50 years old), hypertension (up to 75% of cases), diabetes mellitus (up to 10% of cases), hyperlipidemia, elevated IOP/glaucoma, use of oral contraceptive pill, smoking. Less common predispositions include hypercoagulable states including: polycythemia, multiple myeloma, Waldenström macroglobulinemia, hyperhomocysteinemia, Lupus anticoagulant and antiphospholipid antibodies, dysfibrinogenemia, activated protein C resistance (factor V Leiden mutation), protein C deficiency, protein S deficiency, antithrombin deficiency, prothrombin gene mutation, Factor XII deficiency.

6. Impending CRVO is when a patient is asymptomatic or complains of episodic episodes of blurry vision with venous dilation, retinal hemorrhages, and delayed circulation time. Nonischemic CRVO usually has vision better than 20/200 and minimal capillary nonperfusion. It is the most common form (75%). Ischemic CRVO often has poor vision (worse than 20/200), severe ERG changes, marked RAPD, and significant retinal ischemia (≥10 disk diameters). Patient is more likely to develop ischemic complications. Ten percent of nonischemic patients (absent or mild RAPD) will become ischemic.

7. In older patients, obtain fasting blood glucose, glycosylated hemoglobin and blood pressure measurement to rule out hypertension and diabetes. Consider checking: CBC with differential, platelets, PT/PTT, antinuclear antibody (ANA), rheumatoid factor (RF), ESR, serum protein electrophoresis, lipid profile, hemoglobin electrophoresis (in African American) depending on the clinical situation. In younger patients (<40 years old) and in whom a hypercoagulable state is being considered, check: human immunodeficiency virus (HIV) status, functional protein S assay, functional protein C assay, functional antithrombin III assay (type II heparin-binding mutation), antiphospholipid antibody titer, lupus anticoagulant, anticardiolipin antibody titer (IgG and IgM), homocysteine level (if elevated test for folate, B12, and creatinine), factor XII (Hageman factor) levels, and activated protein C resistance (factor V Leiden mutation PCR assay). If these tests are normal and clinical suspicion for a hypercoagulable state still exists, then order: plasminogen antigen assay, heparin cofactor II assay, thrombin time, reptilase time, and fibrinogen functional assay.

8. 1. Anti-VEGF: intravitreal injections of ranibizumab (Lucentis; CRUISE Study), aflibercept (Eylea; COPERNICUS and GALILEO studies), and bevacizumab (Avastin) have been shown to be beneficial.

   2. Steroids: intravitreal steroid injections were beneficial in the SCORE Study. The dexamethasone implant (Ozurdex) has also been shown to be beneficial in the GENEVA Study. Usually second-line therapy to anti-VEGF agents.

   3. Laser: has not been shown to be beneficial in macular edema due to CRVO; however, panretinal photocoagulation when neovascular complications occur is proven (CVOS conclusion). Early treatment with PRP is not proven.

9. Younger patients (<50 years old) have better prognosis. In nonischemic cases, prognosis is good with improvement in vision in almost 50%. Final vision is related to baseline vision: those better than 20/60 usually do well; those worse than 20/200 do not. Follow patients frequently in first 6–8 months to evaluate for ischemic complications and treat any macular edema. Conversion to ischemic occurs in 15% of cases within 4–6 months, and 30% in 3 years. Risk factors for ischemic complications: (1) Extent of nonperfusion (2) large amounts of retinal hemorrhages (3) short duration of CRVO (4) male.

Index

A

Abetalipoproteinemia, 285–286
ABMD (anterior basement membrane dystrophy), 187–188
Abnormal corneal endothelium, 219–220
AC/A ratio, accommodative esotropia, 119–120
Acanthamoeba keratitis, 189–190
  patient management of, 189–190
Accommodative esotropia, 119–120
Accommodative insufficiency, 19–20
Acid burns, 179–180
Acne rosacea, 191–192
Acquired astigmatism, 212
Acquired hyperopia, 212
Acquired myopia, 212
Acute angle-closure glaucoma, 229–230
  associations of, 229–230
  examination findings of, 229–230
Acute anterior uveitis, 213
  history of, 213–214
Acute dacryoadenitis, 175–176
Acute iritis, 213–214
Acute postoperative endophthalmitis, 221–222
Acute retinal necrosis (ARN), 255–256
Add power
  bifocals, 5–6
  reading glasses, 27–28
Advanced glaucoma, examination of, 237–238
Age, internuclear ophthalmoplegia, 79–80
Age-Related Eye Disease Study (AREDS), 293–294
Age-related macular degeneration (ARMD), exudative, 291–292
AION (anterior ischemic optic neuropathy), 49–50
Alagille's syndrome, 220
Albinism, 277–278
  differential diagnosis of, 277–278
  ocular, 277–278
  oculocutaneous, 278
  other findings of, 277–278
  prognosis of, 277–278
  treatment of, 277–278
Alkali burns, 179–180
Allergic conjunctivitis, 127–128
  characteristics of, 127–128

Allergic conjunctivitis (*Continued*)
  seasonal, 127–128
  treatment of, 127–128
Alstrom's disease, 285–286
Alveolar rhabdomyosarcoma, 137–138
Amblyopia, types of, 117–118
Angle closure, acute, 229–230
Angle recession, 231–232
Angle recession glaucoma, 231–232
Angle-closure glaucoma, 234
  acute, 229–230
Aniridia, 245–246
  associated findings of, 245–246
  etiology of, 245–246
Anisocoria, 51–52
Anisometropia, 117–118
Anisometropic amblyopia, 117–118
Anterior basement membrane dystrophy (ABMD), 187–188
Anterior blepharitis, 191–192
Anterior chamber tap, 201–202
Anterior chamber washout, 233–234
Anterior corneal dystrophies, 187–188
Anterior ischemic optic neuropathy (AION), 49–50
Anterior necrotizing scleritis, 151–152
Anterior scleritis, nodular, 151–152
Anterior segment, of eye, 201–250
Anterior uveitis, 239
  acute, 213
Antibiotic drops, for congenital nasolacrimal duct obstruction, 97–98
Antibiotics
  for chlamydial conjunctivitis, 159–160
  for globe dystopia, 83–84
Antiparasitic therapy, for toxocariasis, 139–140
Anti-vascular endothelial growth factor (VEGF) drugs
  for central retinal vein occlusion, 311–312
  for choroidal neovascularization, 291–292
  for diabetic retinopathy, 281–282
  for presumed ocular histoplasmosis syndrome, 273–274
  for retinal artery macroaneurysm, 309–310
  for retinal vein occlusion, 301–302
Antivirals, 255–256
Antoni A-pattern neurilemmoma, 83–84
Aphakia, contact lenses for, 25
Aphakic glasses, disadvantages of, 25–26

Appositional angle closure, 229–230
AREDS (Age-Related Eye Disease Study), 293–294
ARMD (age-related macular degeneration), 291–292
ARN (acute retinal necrosis), 255–256
Arteriovenous fistula, 91–92
Astigmatic effect, from posterior corneal surface, 39–40
Astigmatism
  acquired, 212
  irregular, 185–186
Atopic keratoconjunctivitis, 127–128
Atrophy, retinal pigment epithelium (RPE), 27
Avonex (interferon β-1a), 65–66
Axenfeld's anomaly, 219–220

B

Band keratopathy, 163–164
Bardet-Biedl syndrome, 285–286
Bartonella henselae infection, 271–272
Basal cell carcinoma (BCC), 177–178
Base-out (BO) prism glasses, 19–20
Bassen-Kornzweig syndrome, 285–286
Batten disease, 285–286
BCC (basal cell carcinoma), 177–178
Benign mixed tumor, treatment of, 175–176
Best disease, 147–148
Bifocals, add power, 5–6
Bilateral congenital cataracts, 113–114
Bilateral involvement, signs of, 79–80
Bilateral uveitis, 207–208
Biopsy
  corneal, 161–162
  for ocular cicatricial pemphigoid, 179–180
  for squamous cell carcinoma, 149–150
Birdshot chorioretinitis, 269–270
Birdshot chorioretinopathy, epidemiology of, 269–270
Blepharitis, 191–192
Blowout fracture, signs of, 75–76
Blurry vision, 223–224
  history of, 181–182
Botryoid rhabdomyosarcoma, 137–138
Brachytherapy, for retinoblastoma, 133–134
Branch retinal vein occlusion, 301–302
BRAVO study, 301–302

Brimonidine, for congenital glaucoma, 95–96
Bullous keratopathy, 235–236
  pseudophakic, 235–236
'Bull's eye' maculopathy, 275–276

C

Callender classification, choroidal malignant melanoma, 289–290
C-ANCA, 181–182
Capillary hemangioma, 111–112
Capsulotomy, laser anterior, 35–36
Cardiac echocardiography, for central retinal artery occlusion, with patent cilioretinal artery, 305–306
Carotid Doppler ultrasound, for central retinal artery occlusion, with patent cilioretinal artery, 305–306
Carotid-cavernous sinus fistula, 91–92
Cataract surgery, 17–18, 113–114, 205–206
  additional information for, 17–18
  causative organism in, 201–202
  characteristic findings of, 221–222
  complications of, 217–218
    risk of, 247–248
  history of, 205–206
  indications for, 247–248
  management of retained material after, 241–242
  risk factors of, 221–222
  treatment of, 217–218
Cataracts, 1–2, 125–126, 165, 217–218
  congenital, 113–114
  epiretinal membrane, 297–298
  mature, 249–250
  posterior polar, 113–114
  posterior subcapsular, 247–248
  radiation therapy, complications of, 289–290
CATT study, 291–292
CBC (complete blood count), 49–50
Cellulitis
  orbital, 57–58, 175–176
  preseptal, 57–58, 175–176
Central retinal artery occlusion, with patent cilioretinal artery, 305–306
Central retinal vein occlusion (CRVO), 311–312
Central serous chorioretinopathy (CSC), 253–254
Chalazion, 175–176
Chalcosis, 261–262
Chandler's syndrome, 220
Chediak-Higashi syndrome, 278
Chemical burns, 179–180
Cherry red spot, 305–306
  differential diagnosis, 305–306

Chiasmal syndrome, 63–64
Chlamydial conjunctivitis, 159–160
Chorioretinitis
  birdshot, 269–270
  toxoplasmosis, 259–260
Chorioretinopathy, birdshot, 269–270
Choristoma, 123–124
Choroidal effusion, 217–218
Choroidal hemangioma, 251–252
Choroidal malignant melanoma, 289–290
Choroidal neovascularization (CNV), 273–274, 291–292
Chromatic aberration, 37–38
Chronic endophthalmitis, 201–202
  characteristic signs of, 201–202
  in ocular larva migrans, 139–140
Chronic progressive external ophthalmoplegia (CPEO), 89–90
  features of, 89–90
Chronic uveitis, 163–164
Chronic vitritis, 257–258
Cicatricial entropion, 155–156
Ciliary body melanoma, 211–212
Cilioretinal artery, 305–306
CIN (conjunctival intraepithelial neoplasia), 153–154
CNV (choroidal neovascularization), 273–274, 291–292
Coats disease, 143–144
  differential diagnosis of, 143–144
Cocaine testing, for Horner's syndrome, 70
Cockayne's syndrome, 285–286
Cogan-Reese syndrome, 220
Cogan's syndrome, 167–168
Collaborative Normal Tension Glaucoma Study (CNTGS), 243–244
Collaborative Ocular Melanoma Study (COMS), 289–290
Coloboma, optic nerve, 93–94
Color vision, testing, 63–64
Complete blood count (CBC), 49–50
Computed tomography (CT), of globe dystopia, 83–84
COMS (Collaborative Ocular Melanoma Study), 289–290
Condensing lenses, 31
Congenital agenesis, 141–142
Congenital cataracts, 113–114
Congenital cloudy cornea, differential diagnosis of, 125–126
Congenital esotropia, 99–100
Congenital glaucoma, 95–96
  breaks in Descemet's membrane and, 125–126
Congenital myogenic ptosis
  characteristics of, 121–122
  prognosis of, 121–122

Congenital nasolacrimal duct obstruction, 97–98
Congenital nystagmus, 101–102
Congenital ptosis, 121–122
Congenital syphilis, 167–168, 207–208
Conjunctiva, lesions, 153–154
Conjunctival injection, 249–250
Conjunctival intraepithelial neoplasia (CIN), 153–154
  biopsy for, 153–154
Conjunctival lymphoid tumor, 173–174
Conjunctival nevus, 183–184
  characteristic of, 183–184
Conjunctival scraping, 159–160
Conjunctivitis
  allergic, 127–128
  chlamydial, 159–160
  etiology of, 159–160
  findings for, 159–160
  follicular, 159–160
  giant papillary, 127–128, 171–172
  membranous, 159–160
  ophthalmia neonatorum, 145–146
  seasonal allergic, 127–128
Contact lenses, 14
  for aphakia, 25
    image magnification with, 25–26
    options for, 25–26
    power of, 25–26
  fitting of, 29
  problems with, 169
Contralateral abducting nystagmus, 79–80
Convergence insufficiency, 19–20
Cornea
  abnormal endothelium, 219–220
  biopsy, 161–162
  edema, 125–126, 235–236
    temporary treatment of, 235–236
  irregular, 15–16
  substances in, 193–194
  topography of, 11–12
    maps for, 13–14
  transplant, 125–126
    Acanthamoeba keratitis, 189–190
Cornea verticillata, 193–194
Corneal astigmatism, 11–12
Corneal dendrite, 197–198
Corneal inflammation, 167–168
Corneal lesion, 65–66
Corneal pachymetry, 165–166
Corneal scars, 125–126
  correction of, 33–34
Corneal staining, 95–96
Corneal thinning, peripheral, 181–182
Corneal topography, diagnosis of, 185–186
  conditions with similar appearance on, 185–186

Corneal ulceration, in allergic conjunctivitis, 127–128
Cortical cataracts, 217–218
Cotton wool spots (CWS), 263–264
  causes of, 263–264
Cranial nerve, examination of, 55–56
Cranial nerve III palsy, 51–52
Cranial nerve VI palsy, 53–54
C-reactive protein (CRP), 49–50
Critical angle, 41–42
CRP (C-reactive protein), 49–50
CT. see Computed tomography (CT).
Culture media, for *Acanthamoeba* keratitis, 189–190
CWS (cotton wool spots), 263–264
Cycloplegic, 233–234
Cycloplegic refraction, 117–118
Cystoid macular edema, 297–298
  pseudophakic, 307–308
Cytomegalovirus (CMV) infections, 255–256

D

Dacryoadenitis, 175–176
  acute, 175–176
DED (dry eye disease), 199–200
Dendritic keratitis, differential diagnosis of, 197–198
Descemet's membrane tears, 125–126
Descemet's stripping automated endothelial keratoplasty (DSAEK), 125–126
Diabetes, in CN 6 palsy, 53–54
Diabetes Control and Complications Trial (DCCT), 281–282
Diabetic macular edema, 1–2
Diabetic retinopathy, 279–280
  differential diagnosis of, 279–280
  findings of, 279–280
  levels of, 281–282
  treatment of, 281–282
Diabetic Retinopathy Study (DRS), 281–282
Diffuse lamellar keratitis (DLK), 7–8
Diffuse large B-cell nonHodgkin's lymphoma, 257–258
Diopters, prism, 21–22, 30
Diplopia, 135–136
  cause of, 73–74
  monocular, 219–220
  patient history of, 53–54, 57–58
  transient, 71–72
  treatment of, 59–60
Dissociated vertical deviation (DVD), surgical procedures for, 99–100
Distance glasses, 23
DLK (diffuse lamellar keratitis), 7–8
Double vision, 53, 105, 135, 219
  eye pain and, 87–88
  in horizontal gaze palsy, 79–80

Down syndrome, 103–104
Droopy eyelid, 51, 69
DRS (Diabetic Retinopathy Study), 281–282
Drusen, 27
  optic nerve head, 47–48
Dry eye disease (DED), 199–200
Dry eyes, 59–60, 179
  questions on, 179–180
DSAEK. see Descemet's stripping automated endothelial keratoplasty (DSAEK).
Duane's retraction syndrome type 3, 141–142
  classification of, 141–142
Duochrome test, 37–38
Dye disappearance test, 97–98
Dysplasias, optic nerve, 93–94
Dystopia, globe, 81–82

E

Early Treatment Diabetic Retinopathy Study (ETDRS), 281–282
  characteristics of, 45–46
Early Treatment of Retinopathy of Prematurity (ETROP) Study, 115–116
Ectopia lentis, 223–224
Ectropion, 195–196
Edema
  cornea, 125–126, 235–236
  cystoid macular, 297–298
    pseudophakic, 307–308
8-ball hyphema, 233–234
Electrocardiogram (EKG), for chronic progressive external ophthalmoplegia, 89–90
Embryonal rhabdomyosarcoma, 137–138
Embryonic fissure, in optic nerve coloboma, 93–94
Empiric topical antibiotic, for ophthalmia neonatorum conjunctivitis, 145–146
Endophthalmitis
  acute postoperative, 221–222
  chronic, 201–202
  P.acnes, 201–202
  reduce rate of, 221–222
Endophthalmitis Vitrectomy Study (EVS), 221–222
Endothelium, abnormal corneal, 219–220
Entropion, 155–156
  cicatricial, 155–156
  involutional, 155–156
  spastic, 155–156
Enucleation, for retinoblastoma, 133–134
Epiretinal membrane (ERM), 297–298
Episcleritis, 151–152
Epithelial basement membrane dystrophy (EBMD), 187–188
Epithelioid cells, 289–290

ERM (epiretinal membrane), 297–298
Erythrocyte sedimentation rate (ESR), 49–50
Esotropia (ET), 53–54, 99–100
  accommodative, 119–120
  congenital, 99–100
ESR (erythrocyte sedimentation rate), 49–50
Essential iris atrophy, 220
ETDRS (Early Treatment Diabetic Retinopathy Study), 281–282
Ethambutol, causing toxic optic neuropathy, 85–86
ETROP (Early Treatment of Retinopathy of Prematurity) Study, 115–116
EVS (Endophthalmitis Vitrectomy Study), 221–222
External disease/adnexa, 149–200
Extraocular motility, 77–78
Exudative age-related macular, degeneration, 291–292
Exudative retinal detachment, 251–252
Eye disorders, in Down syndrome, 103–104
Eye examination
  in Down syndrome, 103–104
  for idiopathic orbital inflammatory disease, 87–88
  for retrobulbar optic neuritis, 65–66
  for thyroid-related ophthalmopathy, 59–60
Eye pain, 65–66, 151
  additional questions for, 151–152
  differential diagnosis, 87–88
  myopia and, 189
    questions for, 189–190
Eyelid, droopy, 51, 69
Eyelid capillary hemangioma, 111–112
Eyes
  anatomic factors of, 203–204
  deterioration of vision in, 223–224
  red, 91–92
  surgery for, 217–218
Eyestrain, 19

F

Fabry's disease, cornea verticillata and, 193–194
Flat bleb, in advanced glaucoma, 237–238
  differential diagnosis of, 237–238
Flexner-Wintersteiner rosette, 131–132
Floppy eyelid syndrome, 157–158
Fluorescein angiogram
  for 'bull's eye' maculopathy, 275–276
  for central retinal artery occlusion, 305–306
  for central retinal vein occlusion, 311–312
  for central serous chorioretinopathy, 253–254
  for diabetic retinopathy, 279–280

Fluorescein angiogram (*Continued*)
   for epiretinal membrane, 295–296
   for exudative age-related macular
      degeneration, 291–292
   for exudative retinal detachment, 251–252
   of iris, 215–216
   for macular hole, 265–266
   for multiple evanescent white dot
      syndrome, 303–304
   for presumed ocular histoplasmosis
      syndrome, 273–274
   for pseudophakic cystoid macular edema,
      307–308
   for retinal artery macroaneurysm, 309–310
   for retinal vein occlusion, 301–302
   for Stargardt disease, 129–130
Follicular conjunctivitis, 159–160
Foster-Kennedy syndrome, 49–50
Fuchs endothelial dystrophy, 165–166
Fuchs heterochromic iridocyclitis, 239–240
Functional visual loss, 67–68
Fundus autofluorescence, for multiple
      evanescent white dot syndrome,
      303–304
Fungal keratitis, 161–162
Fungal ulcers, 161–162

G

Gaze palsy, horizontal, 79–80
GCA (giant cell arteritis), 227–228
Generalized fundus hypopigmentation,
      277–278
Generous optic cups, 243
Genetics
   of retinoblastoma, 132
   of Stargardt disease, 129–130
Geneva lens clock, 23–24
GENEVA (Global Evaluation of Implantable
      Dexamethasone in Retinal Vein
      Occlusion with Macular Edema)
      study, 301–302
Giant cell arteritis (GCA), 49–50, 227–228
Giant papillary conjunctivitis (GPC),
      127–128, 171–172
   causes of, 171–172
   differential diagnosis of, 169–170
   treatment for, 171–172
Glare, 10
Glasses
   for astigmatism, 11–12
   difficulty adjusting to, 23–24
   reading, 19
Glaucoma, 205–206
   angle recession, 231–232
   angle-closure, 234. *see also* Angle-closure
      glaucoma.
   congenital, 95–96

Glaucoma (*Continued*)
   malignant, 237
   mechanism of, 209–210
   neovascular, 233–234
   optic nerve head drusen and, 47–48
   pigmentary, 209–210
   surgery for, 163
   trabeculectomy, 231–232
Global Evaluation of Implantable
      Dexamethasone in Retinal Vein
      Occlusion with Macular Edema
      (GENEVA) Study, 301–302
Globe displacement, 135–136
Globe dystopia, 81–82
Goldenhar's syndrome, in limbal dermoid,
      123–124
Goldmann-style lenses, 42
Gomez-Morales staging, of Coats disease,
      143–144
Gonioscopy, 205–206
   indentation, 229–230
   lenses, 41–42
Goniotomy, for congenital glaucoma, 95–96
GPC (giant papillary conjunctivitis),
      171–172
Granuloma
   localized, 139–140
   peripheral, 139–140
Granulomatous uveitis, 259–260
Graves' disease, 59–60

H

Haab's striae, 95–96
Hagberg-Santavuori syndrome, 285–286
Halos, 165
Head, position of, in left superior oblique
      palsy, 105–106
Headache, 19, 51–52
Hemorrhages
   intraretinal, 109
   suprachoroidal, 217–218
Heritable disease, albinism as, 277–278
Hermansky-Pudlak syndrome, 278
Herpes simplex virus (HSV) epithelial
      keratitis, 197–198
Herpes simplex virus (HSV) infections,
      255–256
Herpes simplex virus (HSV) keratitis,
      189–190
Herpes simplex virus (HSV) stromal keratitis,
      treatment of, 197–198
Herpes zoster ophthalmicus (HZO), 227–228
Herpes zoster virus (HZV) infections,
      227–228, 255–256
Heterochromia, iris, 239–240
High index lenses, 13–14
Histoplasma capsulatum infection, 273–274

History, of myasthenia gravis, 71–72
HLA-A29, birdshot chorioretinitis and,
      269–270
HLA-B27
   disorders associated with, 213–214
   iritis associated with, 213–214
Holladay R formula, 44
Homer-Wright rosette, 131–134
Homocystinuria, 224
Horizontal gaze palsy, 79–80
Horner's syndrome, 55–56, 69–70
   etiologies of, 69–70
   pharmacologic testing for, 69–70
Horner-Trantas dot, 127–128
Horseshoe, retinal tears, 267–268
Hutchinson's sign, 227–228
Hydrops, 185–186
Hydroxyamphetamine, for Horner's
      syndrome, 70
Hydroxychloroquine retinal toxicity,
      275–276
Hyperlysinemia, 224
Hyperopia, 19–20, 117–118
   acquired, 212
Hyphema, 233–234
   8-ball, 233–234
Hysteria, 67–68
HZO (herpes zoster ophthalmicus),
      227–228

I

ICE syndrome, 219–220
Idiopathic intracranial hypertension (IIH),
      73–74
Idiopathic orbital inflammatory disease,
      87–88
IFIS (intraoperative floppy iris syndrome),
      205–206
IIH (idiopathic intracranial hypertension),
      73–74
Image displacement, 3–4
Image jump, 3–4
Imaging, for multiple cranial nerve palsies,
      55–56
Indentation gonioscopy, 229–230
Indirect ophthalmoscope, 31–32
Indocyanine green angiography (ICG)
   for central serous chorioretinopathy,
      253–254
   for exudative age-related macular
      degeneration, 291–292
   for exudative retinal detachment, 251–252
   for multiple evanescent white dot
      syndrome, 303–304
Induced myopia, 21–22
   management of, 21–22
Inert intraocular foreign body, 261–262

Infections, in interstitial keratitis, 167, 168 *see also specific infections.*
Infectious uveitis, 257–258
Intacs, 8
Interferon β-1a (Avonex), 65–66
Intermittent photopsias, 289
Internuclear ophthalmoplegia, 79–80
Interstitial keratitis, 167–168
    treatment for, 167–168
Intraocular foreign body (IOFB), 261–262
Intraocular lenses (IOLs)
    exchange, 36
    phakic. *see* Phakic intraocular lenses.
    piggyback
        considerations for, 43–44
        power of, 43–44
    repositioning of, 225–226
    secondary, 203–204
    subluxed, 225–226
    sulcus, 203–204
Intraocular pressure (IOP)
    high, 209–210
    in optic nerve head drusen, 47–48
Intraoperative floppy iris syndrome (IFIS), 205–206
Intraretinal hemorrhages, 109
Involutional entropion, 155–156
IOFB (intraocular foreign body), 261–262
IOLs. *see* Intraocular lenses (IOLs).
IOP. *see* Intraocular pressure (IOP).
Iris
    essential atrophy, 219–220
    heterochromia, 239–240
        etiology of, 239–240
    neovascularization, 233–234
    progressive atrophy, 220
Iris malignant melanoma, 215–216
Iris nevus (Cogan-Reese) syndrome, 220, 240
Iritis, 95–96, 239–240
    acute, 213–214
    anterior segment signs of, 239–240
    associated with HLA-B27, 213–214
    color changes, 213–214
    fluorescein angiogram for, 215–216
    nongranulomatous, 213–214
    possible complications of, 213–214
    rebound, intraocular inflammation due to, 201–202
Irregular astigmatism, keratoconus and, 185–186
Irritated eyes, history of, 155–158
Irvine-Gass syndrome, 307–308
Ischemic isolated mononeuropathy, 53–54
Isolated palsy, 105–106
Itchy eyes, questions on, 159–160

J

Junctional scotoma, 63–64

K

Kassabach-Merritt syndrome, 111–112
Kearns-Sayre syndrome, 89–90, 285–286
    features of, 89–90
Keratitis
    diffuse lamellar, 7–8
    fungal, 161–162
    herpes simplex virus, 189–190
    interstitial, 167–168
    microbial, 161–162
    patient management for, 161–162
Keratoacanthoma, 149–150
Keratoconjunctivitis
    atopic, 127–128
    vernal, 127–128
Keratoconus (KC), 185–186
Keratometer, 39–40
    limitations of, 39–40
Keratopathy
    band, 163–164
    bullous, 235–236
    pseudophakic bullous, 235–236
Keratotomy
    photorefractive, 13–14
    radial
        examination for, 9–10
        symptoms and treatment options for, 9–10
Kestenbaum procedure, for congenital nystagmus, 101–102
Kestenbaum's rule, 27–28
Koeppe-style lenses, 42
Kruckenberg spindle, 209–210

L

Laboratory tests
    of birdshot chorioretinitis, 269–270
    of central retinal vein occlusion, 311–312
    of cotton wool spots, 263–264
    of granulomatous uveitis, 259–260
    of neuroretinitis, 271–272
    of retinal vein occlusion, 301–302
Lacrimal gland tumors, 175–176
Laser anterior capsulotomy, 36
Laser iridoplasty, 229–230
Laser photocoagulation, for diabetic retinopathy, 281–282
Laser trabeculoplasty, 231–232
Laser treatment
    for central retinal vein occlusion, 311–312
    for presumed ocular histoplasmosis syndrome, 273–274
    for retinal vein occlusion, 301–302

Laser-assisted in situ keratomileusis (LASIK)
    for astigmatism, 185
    complications of, 7–8
    for myopia, 185
LASIK. *see* Laser-assisted in situ keratomileusis (LASIK).
Laurence-Moon syndrome, 285–286
Leber's hereditary optic neuropathy (LHON), 61–62
    characteristic findings of, 61–62
Leber's idiopathic stellate neuroretinitis, 271–272
Left hypertropia, 105
Left superior oblique palsy, 105–106
Lens extraction, surgical techniques for, 223–224
Lenses
    condensing, 31
    intraocular. *see* Intraocular lenses (IOLs).
    minus, 21–22
Lens-induced glaucoma, 249–250
Leukocoria, 131–132
LHON (Leber's hereditary optic neuropathy), 61–62
Limbal dermoid, 123–124
    treatment of, 123–124
Lipofuscinosis, neuronal ceroid, 285–286
Localized granuloma, in ocular larva migrans, 139–140
Low-vision aids, 27–28
    for exudative age-related macular, degeneration, 293–294
Lumbar puncture, for idiopathic intracranial hypertension, 73–74
Lymphoid tumor, conjunctival, 173–174

M

Macular degeneration, 27
Macular edema, cystoid, 297–298
Macular hole, stage 3, 265–266
Maculopathy, 'bull's eye', 275–276
Magnification, types of, 31–32
Malignant glaucoma, 237
    anterior chamber appearance in, 237–238
    treatment of, 237–238
Malignant melanoma, 183–184
    choroidal, 289–290
    ciliary body, 211–212
    diagnosis of, 215–216
Malingering, 67–68
Map-dot-fingerprint (MDF) dystrophy, 187–188
Marfan's syndrome, 223–224
Marginal keratolysis, 181–182
Maximal levator resection, for congenital myogenic ptosis, 121–122

Medial canthus, 177–178

Medial longitudinal fasciculus, 79–80

Medial rectus muscle, 99–100

Medial rectus palsy, internuclear ophthalmoplegia and, 79–80

Medical history
   of congenital nasolacrimal duct obstruction, 97–98
   of corneal scars and cataract, 125–126
   of diplopia, 135–136
   of trauma, 109–110

Medications, associated with idiopathic intracranial hypertension, 73–74

Meesmann dystrophy, 187–188

Meibomian gland, 191–192

Meibomian gland dysfunction (MGD), 191–192
   treatment for, 191–192

Melanocytoma, 215–216

Melanoma, malignant. *see* Malignant melanoma.

Melanosis, primary acquired, 183–184
   with atypia, treatment and prognosis of, 183–184
   indication for biopsy of, 183–184

Membranous conjunctivitis, 159–160

Mesodermal dysgenesis syndrome, 219–220

Metastases, malignant melanoma, 289–290

Methylprednisolone, for retrobulbar optic neuritis, 65–66

MG (myasthenia gravis), 71–72

Microbial keratitis, 161–162

Minus lenses, 21–22

Miotic pupil, differential diagnosis of, 69–70

Miotics, 229–230

Mooren's ulcer, 181–182

Motor nystagmus, 101–102

Mucor infection, 57–58

Mucormycosis, 58

Multiple cranial nerve palsies, 55–56

Multiple evanescent white dot syndrome (MEWDS), 303–304

Myasthenia gravis (MG), 71–72
   chronic progressive external ophthalmoplegia and, 89–90
   internuclear ophthalmoplegia and, 79–80

Mydriatic pupil, differential diagnosis of, 69–70

Myopia
   acquired, 212
   decreased, 1–2
   eye pain and, 189
   induced, 21–22
      management of, 21–22
   surgical correction for, 7–8

Myopic refractive outcome, 35–36

N

NAION (nonarteritic anterior ischemic optic neuropathy), 49–50

Nasolacrimal duct obstruction (NLDO), 95–96
   congenital, 97–98

Nasolacrimal irrigation, 97–98

Nd:YAG laser posterior capsulotomy, 225

Neovascular glaucoma (NVG), 233–234

Neovascularization, iris, 233–234

Neuroimaging
   for cranial nerve III palsy, 51–52
   for idiopathic intracranial hypertension, 73–74
   for junctional scotoma, 63–64
   for retinoblastoma, 131–132
   for right homonymous inferior quadrantic scotomas, 77–78

Neuronal ceroid lipofuscinosis, 285–286

Neuro-ophthalmology/orbit, 47–94

Neuroretinitis, 271–272

Neurosyphilis, 207–208

Nevus
   conjunctival, 183–184
      characteristic of, 183–184
      differential diagnosis of, 215–216

Nodular anterior scleritis, 151–152

Nonarteritic anterior ischemic optic neuropathy (NAION), 49–50

Nongranulomatous iritis, 213–214

NonHodgkin's lymphoma, diffuse large B-cell, 257–258

Noninfectious uveitis, 257–258

NSAID drops, for pseudophakic cystoid macular edema, 308

NSAIDs, for scleritis, 151–152

Nuclear sclerotic cataracts, 217–218

Nutritional optic neuropathy, 85–86

NVG (neovascular glaucoma), 233–234

Nystagmus
   congenital, 101–102
   motor, 101–102

O

Oblique muscle overaction, 107–108

OCP (ocular cicatricial pemphigoid), 179–180

OCT. *see* Optical coherence tomography (OCT).

Ocular albinism, 277–278

Ocular cicatricial pemphigoid (OCP), 179–180

Ocular colobomas, 93–94

Ocular history, 207–208

Ocular ischemia, 233–234

Ocular larva migrans, 139–140

Ocular misalignment, 51–52

Ocular motility testing, 53

Ocular testing, 211–212

Oculocutaneous albinism, 278

One-and-a-half syndrome, 79–80

ONTT (Optic Neuritis Treatment Trial), 65–66

Ophthalmia neonatorum conjunctivitis, 145–146

Ophthalmopathy, thyroid-related, 59–60

Ophthalmoscope, indirect, 31–32

Optic cupping, 231

Optic disc
   pallor, 63–64
   swelling, 73–74

Optic nerve
   coloboma, 93–94
   dysplasias, 93–94

Optic nerve head drusen (pseudopapilledema), 47–48
   complications of, 47
   diagnosis of, 47–48
   pathophysiology of, 47–48

Optic neuritis, retrobulbar, 65–66

Optic Neuritis Treatment Trial (ONTT), 65–66

Optic neuropathies
   differential diagnosis of, 85–86
   hereditary or acquired, 61–62
   history for, 85–86
   nutritional, 85–86
   toxic, 85–86

Optical coherence tomography (OCT)
   for central retinal artery occlusion, 305–306
   for central retinal vein occlusion, 311–312
   for central serous chorioretinopathy, 253–254
   for cystoid macular edema, pseudophakic, 307–308
   for diabetic retinopathy, 279–280
   for epiretinal membrane, 295–296
   for exudative age-related macular degeneration, 291–292
   for exudative retinal detachment, 251–252
   for macular hole, 265–266
   for multiple evanescent white dot syndrome, 303–304

Optics/refraction, 1–46

Oral antivirals, 227–228

Orbital apex syndrome, *Mucor* infection and, 57–58

Orbital cellulitis, 57–58, 135–136, 175–176

Orbital floor fracture, 75–76
   treatment of, 75–76

Orbital mass, globe displacement in, 135–136

Orthoptic exercises, 19–20

P

PAM (primary acquired melanosis), 183–184
Papilledema, 73–74
Parietal lobe, lesion in, 77–78
Parks-Bielschowsky 3-step test, 105–106
PBK (pseudophakic bullous keratopathy), 235–236
PDS (pigment dispersion syndrome), 209–210
PDT. see Photodynamic therapy (PDT).
Pediatric floor fractures, 75–76
Peripheral corneal thinning, 181–182
Peripheral granuloma, in ocular larva migrans, 139–140
Peripheral posterior cortical/subcapsular cataract, additional history of, 231–232
Periventricular white matter demyelinating lesions, 65–66
Peter's anomaly, 220
PG (pigmentary glaucoma), 209–210
Phacoemulsification, 217–218, 223–224
Phacolytic glaucoma, 249–250
    characteristics of, 249–250
Phakic intraocular lenses, 14
    complications of, 13–14
Phenylephrine, for differentiating scleritis and episcleritis, 151–152
PHN (postherpetic neuralgia), 227–228
Photocoagulation, for retinoblastoma, 133–134
Photodynamic therapy (PDT)
    for central serous chorioretinopathy, 253–254
    for choroidal neovascularization, 291–292
    for presumed ocular histoplasmosis syndrome, 273–274
Photophobia, treatment of, 245–246
Photopsias, intermittent, 289
Photorefractive keratotomy (PRK), 13–14
Piggyback intraocular lenses, 36
    considerations for, 43–44
    power of, 43–44
Pigment dispersion syndrome (PDS), 209–210
Pigmentary glaucoma (PG), 209–210
Pinhole, 34, 45
    optimal size of, 45–46
Pinhole vision, 21–22
PIOL (primary intraocular lymphoma), 257–258
Pisciform flecks, 129–130
Plateau-iris syndrome, 229–230
    pathophysiology of, 229–230
Pleomorphic rhabdomyosarcoma, 137–138
Plus disease, 115–116

POHS (presumed ocular histoplasmosis syndrome), 273–274
Posterior capsule tear/rupture, 113–114, 241–242
Posterior polar cataract, 113–114
    treatment of, 113–114
Posterior scleritis, 151–152
Posterior segment, of eye, 251–312
Posterior subcapsular cataracts, 247–248
    diagnosis of, 247–248
Posterior vitreous detachment, 267–268
Postherpetic neuralgia (PHN), 227–228
Postoperative endophthalmitis, acute, 221–222
Prednisone
    for giant cell arteritis, 49–50
    for retrobulbar optic neuritis, 65–66
Presbyopia, 3–4
    decreased, 1–2
    options for, 3–4
Preseptal cellulitis, 57–58, 175–176
Presumed ocular histoplasmosis syndrome (POHS), 273–274
Primary acquired melanosis (PAM), 183–184
    with atypia, treatment and prognosis of, 183–184
    indication for biopsy of, 183–184
Primary intraocular lymphoma (PIOL), 257–258
Prince rule, 6
Prism adaptation test, 107–108
Prism diopters, 21–22, 30
Prism dissociation, 6
Prisms, measurement with, 21–22
PRK (photorefractive keratotomy), 13–14
Progressive base-out prism, 107–108
Progressive hyperopic shift, 10
Progressive iris atrophy, 220
Progressive lenses, advantages of, 3–4
Propionibacterium acnes infection, 201
Proptosis, 59–60, 69–70
Provocative tests, for acute angle-closure glaucoma, 229–230
Pseudoexfoliation syndrome (PXS), 205–206
    etiologies of, 225–226
Pseudo-Foster-Kennedy syndrome, 49–50
Pseudopapilledema, 47–48
Pseudophakic bullous keratopathy (PBK), 235–236
Pseudophakic cystoid macular edema, 307–308
Ptosis, 51–52, 89–90
    asymmetric, 71–72
    congenital, 121–122
Pupils, in idiopathic intracranial hypertension, 73–74

Pupil-sparing third nerve palsy, isolated, 51–52
PXS (pseudoexfoliation syndrome), 205–206

Q

Quadrantic scotomas, right homonymous inferior, 77–78
Quinolones, toxicity, 275–276

R

Radial keratotomy (RK) surgery
    examination for, 9–10
    symptoms and treatment options for, 9–10
Radiation retinopathy, 289–290
Radiation therapy, complications of, 289–290
Reading glasses, 19
    add power of, 27–28
Rebound iritis, intraocular inflammation due to, 201–202
Reese-Ellsworth classification, 133–134
Refraction, cycloplegic, 117–118
Refractive accommodative esotropia, 119–120
Refractive error, 211–212
Refractive lens exchange (RLE), 13–14
Refractive outcome, myopic, 35–36
Refractive surprise, 35–36
Refsum's disease, 285–286
Reis-Bucklers dystrophy, 187–188
Respiratory infection, 159–160
Retinal artery macroaneurysm, 309–310
Retinal detachment
    exudative, 251–252
    repair, 21
Retinal exams, for stage 3 retinopathy of prematurity, 115–116
Retinal ischemia, laser photocoagulation for, 233–234
Retinal necrosis, 255–256
Retinal pigment epithelium (RPE) atrophy, 27
Retinal tears, 267–268
    horseshoe, 267–268
Retinal vascular occlusions, *Mucor* infection and, 57–58
Retinal vein occlusion (RVO), 301–302
Retinitis, viral, 255–256
Retinitis pigmentosa (RP), 283–284
    inversus, 285–286
    sector, 285–286
    sine pigmento, 285–286
Retinitis punctata albescens, 285–286
Retinoblastoma, 131–132

Retinopathy, radiation, 289–290

Retinopathy of prematurity (ROP), 109–110, 115–116

    stage 3, 115–116

Retinoscopy, streak, 15–16

Retrobulbar block, 217–218

Retrobulbar optic neuritis, 65–66

Reverse pupillary block, 209–210

RGP. *see* Rigid gas permeable (RGP) contact lenses.

Rhabdomyosarcoma, 137–138

    alveolar, 137–138

    botryoid, 137–138

    embryonal, 137–138

    pleomorphic, 137–138

Rhegmatogenous retinal detachment, 251–252, 267–268

Rheumatoid arthritis, scleromalacia perforans and, 151–152

Rieger's anomaly, 220

Rieger's syndrome, 220

Right homonymous inferior quadrantic scotomas, 77–78

Rigid gas permeable (RGP) contact lenses, 29–30, 203

ROP (retinopathy of prematurity), 109–110, 115–116

RP (retinitis pigmentosa), 283–284

RPE (retinal pigment epithelium) atrophy, 27

Rubeosis, 233–234

RVO (retinal vein occlusion), 301–302

S

Sagging, in entropion, 155–156

Salmon patch, 173–174

Scars, corneal. *see* Corneal scars.

Scissoring reflex, 15–16

Scleral buckle, 21

Scleral-sutured intraocular lenses, 203–204

Scleritis, 151–152

    nodular anterior, 151–152

    posterior, 151–152

Scleromalacia perforans, 151–152

Scotoma, junctional, 63–64

Seasonal allergic conjunctivitis, 127–128

Sebaceous cell carcinoma, 177–178

Sebaceous gland carcinoma, 149–150

Secondary intraocular lenses, 203–204

Sector retinitis pigmentosa, 285–286

Shaken baby syndrome, 109–110

Siderosis, 261–262

Sigelman staging, of Coats disease, 143–144

Skin cancer, 177–178

    history of, 183–184

Slit-lamp examination, 231–232

Snapback test, for entropion, 155–156

Snellen acuity, 45–46

Snellen notation, 45–46

Soft contact lens (SCL), fitting for, 29–30

Spasmus nutans, 101–102

Spastic entropion, 155–156

Specular microscopy, 165–166

Spindle A cells, 289–290

Spindle B cells, 289–290

Squamous cell carcinoma, 149–150

    treatment for, 149–150, 153–154

Stains, for *Acanthamoeba* keratitis, 189–190

Staphylococcus aureus infection, acute postoperative endophthalmitis, 221–222

Starburst, 10

Stargardt disease, 129–130

    prognosis of, 129–130

Steroids

    for central retinal vein occlusion, 311–312

    for diabetic retinopathy, 281–282

    for giant cell arteritis, 49–50

    for idiopathic orbital inflammatory disease, 87–88

    for retinal vein occlusion, 301–302

Stevens-Johnson syndrome, 179–180

Strabismus, 71–72

Strabismus surgery, 99–100

Streak retinoscopy, 15–16

Subconjunctival hemorrhage, 75

Subjective manifest refraction, 5–6

Sulcus intraocular lens, 203–204, 226

Sulfite oxidase deficiency, 224

Sunset syndrome, 225–226

Superior tarsal conjunctival papillae, 157–158

Suprachoroidal hemorrhage, 217–218

Surgery

    for corneal scar correction, 33–34

    for glaucoma, 163

    indications of, for orbital floor fracture, 75–76

    for myopia, 7–8

    presumed ocular histoplasmosis syndrome, 273–274

Surgical excision, for globe dystopia, 83–84

Swollen left upper eyelid, questions on, 175–176

Symblepharon, 179–180

Synechial angle closure, 229

Syphilis, congenital, 207–208

Systemic diseases, eye pain and, 87–88

Systemic lymphoma, risk of, 173–174

Systemic steroids, for capillary hemangioma, 111–112

T

TASS (toxic anterior segment syndrome), 221–222

Tensilon test, 71–72

Tension glaucoma, normal, 243–244

Terrien's marginal degeneration, 181–182

Thiel-Behnke dystrophy, 187–188

Thyroid-related ophthalmopathy (TRO), 59–60

Tolosa-Hunt syndrome, 87–88

Topical cycloplegic, for iris heterochromia, 239–240

Topical medications, for congenital glaucoma, 95–96

Topical steroids, 233–234

    inflammation with, 235–236

    for iris heterochromia, 239–240

Topography maps, corneal, 13–14

Total internal reflection, 41–42

Toxic anterior segment syndrome (TASS), 221–222

Toxic optic neuropathy, 85–86

Toxicity, hydroxychloroquine, 275–276

Toxocara canis, 139–140

Toxocara cati, 139–140

Toxocariasis, 139–140

Toxoplasmosis chorioretinitis, 259–260

Trabeculectomy, for glaucoma, 231–232

Trabeculotomy, for congenital glaucoma, 95–96

Transient diplopia, 71–72

Transplant, cornea, 125–126

Trauma, 105–106, 109–110

    treatment of, 109–110

Treponema pallidum, 207–208

    ocular findings of, 207–208

Triamcinolone, 241–242

TRO (thyroid-related ophthalmopathy), 59–60

True albinism, 278

Tumor(s)

    conjunctival lymphoid, 173–174

    extent of, 211–212

    lacrimal gland, 175–176

20D lens, 31–32

U

Uhthoff's symptom, 65–66

UKPDS (United Kingdom Prospective Diabetes Study), 281–282

Ultrasound, for choroidal malignant melanoma, 289–290

United Kingdom Prospective Diabetes Study (UKPDS), 281–282

Upper eyelid, everted, 157–158, 169–170

Usher's syndrome, 285–286

Uveitis
    anterior. *see* Anterior uveitis.
    bilateral, 207–208
    chronic, 163–164
    granulomatous, 259–260
    infectious, 257–258
    noninfectious, 257–258

V

Vernal keratoconjunctivitis (VKC),
        127–128
    self-limited, 127–128
Viral retinitis, 255–256
Viroptic, 189
    toxicity, 189–190

Vision
    in eyelid capillary hemangioma, 111–112
    gradual decrease in, history of, 165–166
    loss
        functional, 67–68
        history of, 61–62
        in Leber's hereditary optic neuropathy,
            61–62
        "recover", 67–68
Vision tests, 67–68
Visual acuity, in esotropia, 99–100
Visual field (VF)
    defect, in optic nerve head drusen,
        47–48
    exam, for optic neuropathies, 85–86
    testing, 63–64

Vitamin deficiencies, in nutritional optic
        neuropathy, 85–86
Vitelliform macular dystrophy, 147–148
Vitiliginous chorioretinitis. *see* Birdshot
        chorioretinitis.
Vitritis, chronic, 257–258
V-pattern exotropia (XT), 107–108

W

Watery eye, 97
Watzke-Allen sign, in macular hole, 265–266
Wegener's granulomatosis, 181–182
Weill-Marchesani syndrome, 224
Werner classification, of thyroid-related
        ophthalmopathy, 59–60

Index of Cases

Optics/Refraction (Chapter 1)

1   Overcorrected Myopia with Presbyopia   1
2   Bifocals   3
3   Refraction Technique   5
4   LASIK Complications   7
5   Radial Keratotomy Complications   9
6   Astigmatism   11
7   Refractive Surgery Options   13
8   Retinoscopy   15
9   Anisometropia   17
10   Convergence Insufficiency   19
11   Prisms   21
12   Base Curve   23
13   Lens Effectivity   25
14   Low Vision Aids   27
15   Contact Lens Fitting   29
16   Magnification   31
17   Corneal Scar Management   33
18   IOL Surprise   35
19   Duochrome Test   37
20   Keratometer   39
21   Gonioscopy and Total Internal Reflection   41
22   Piggyback IOL   43
23   Visual Acuity and Pinhole   45

Neuro-ophthalmology/Orbit (Chapter 2)

24   Optic Nerve Drusen   47
25   Anterior Ischemic Optic Neuropathy   49
26   Cranial Nerve 3 Palsy   51
27   Cranial Nerve 6 Palsy   53
28   Multiple Cranial Nerve Palsies   55
29   Orbital Cellulitis   57
30   Thyroid-related Ophthalmopathy   59
31   Leber's Hereditary Optic Neuropathy   61
32   Junction Scotoma   63
33   Optic Neuritis   65
34   Functional Visual Loss   67
35   Anisocoria   69
36   Myasthenia Gravis   71
37   Idiopathic Intracranial Hypertension   73
38   Orbital Fracture   75
39   Homonymous Visual Field Defect   77
40   Internuclear Ophthalmoplegia   79
41   Orbital Tumors   81

42   Toxic/Nutritional Optic Neuropathy   85
43   Idiopathic Orbital Inflammatory Disease (Orbital Pseudotumor)   87
44   Chronic Progressive External Ophthalmoplegia   89
45   Carotid-Cavernous Sinus Fistula   91
46   Optic Nerve Coloboma   93

Pediatric Ophthalmology/Strabismus (Chapter 3)

47   Congenital Glaucoma   95
48   Nasolacrimal Duct Obstruction   97
49   Esotropia   99
50   Nystagmus   101
51   Down Syndrome   103
52   Superior Oblique Palsy   105
53   Exotropia (V-pattern)   107
54   Shaken Baby Syndrome   109
55   Capillary Hemangioma   111
56   Congenital Cataract   113
57   Retinopathy of Prematurity   115
58   Anisometropic Amblyopia   117
59   AC/A ratio   119
60   Congenital Ptosis   121
61   Limbal Dermoid   123
62   Corneal Birth Trauma   125
63   Vernal Keratoconjunctivitis   127
64   Stargardt Disease   129
65   Leukocoria/Retinoblastoma   131
66   Rhabdomyosarcoma   135
67   Toxocariasis   139
68   Duane's Retraction Syndrome   141
69   Coats Disease   143
70   Ophthalmia Neonatorum   145
71   Best Disease   147

External Disease/Adnexa (Chapter 4)

72   Keratoacanthoma   149
73   Scleritis   151
74   Conjunctival Intraepithelial Neoplasia   153
75   Entropion   155
76   Floppy Eyelid Syndrome   157
77   Chlamydial Conjunctivitis   159
78   Fungal Keratitis   161
79   Band Keratopathy   163
80   Fuchs Corneal Dystrophy   165
81   Interstitial Keratitis   167
82   Giant Papillary Conjunctivitis   169

83   Conjunctival Lymphoid Tumor   173
84   Lacrimal Gland Tumor/Dacryoadenitis   175
85   Basal Cell Carcinoma of Eyelid   177
86   Cicatrizing Ocular Surface Disease   179
87   Peripheral Ulcerative Keratitis   181
88   Primary Acquired Melanosis   183
89   Keratoconus   185
90   Epithelial Basement Membrane Dystrophy/Recurrent Erosion Syndrome   187
91   *Acanthamoeba* Keratitis   189
92   Meibomian Gland Dysfunction/Acne Rosacea   191
93   Cornea Verticillata   193
94   Ectropion   195
95   HSV Keratitis   197
96   Dry Eye Disease   199

Anterior Segment (Chapter 5)

97   *P. acnes* Chronic Endophthalmitis   201
98   Secondary IOL Options   203
99   Pseudoexfoliation Syndrome/IFIS   205
100   Syphilis   207
101   Pigment Dispersion Syndrome   209
102   Ciliary Body Melanoma   211
103   HLA-B27 associated Iritis   213
104   Iris Melanoma   215
105   Cataract Workup and Complications   217
106   ICE Syndromes   219
107   Acute Postoperative Endophthalmitis   221
108   Ectopia Lentis   223
109   Dislocated IOL   225
110   Herpes Zoster Ophthalmicus   227
111   Angle-closure Glaucoma/Plateau Iris Syndrome   229
112   Angle Recession Glaucoma   231
113   Rubeosis/Hyphema   233
114   Pseudophakic Bullous Keratopathy   235
115   Trabeculectomy Complication (Flat Bleb)   237
116   Fuchs Heterochromic Iridocyclitis   239
117   Retained Lens Fragment after Cataract Surgery   241
118   Normal Tension Glaucoma   243

119 Aniridia   245
120 Posterior Subcapsular Cataract   247
121 Phacolytic Glaucoma   249

Posterior Segment (Chapter 6)
122 Exudative Retinal Detachment   251
123 Central Serous Chorioretinopathy   253
124 Acute Retinal Necrosis   255
125 Lymphoma   257
126 Toxoplasmosis Chorioretinitis   259
127 Intraocular Foreign Body   261

128 Cotton Wool Spots   263
129 Macular Hole   265
130 Posterior Vitreous Detachment/ Retinal Tear   267
131 Birdshot Retinochoroidopathy   269
132 Neuroretinitis   271
133 Presumed Ocular Histoplasmosis Syndrome   273
134 Bull's Eye Maculopathy   275
135 Ocular Albinism   277
136 Diabetic Retinopathy   279

137 Retinitis Pigmentosa   283
138 Choroidal Malignant Melanoma   289
139 Age-related Macular Degeneration   291
140 Epiretinal Membrane   295
141 Branch Retinal Vein Occlusion   299
142 Multiple Evanescent White Dot Syndrome   303
143 Central Retinal Artery Occlusion   305
144 Cystoid Macular Edema   307
145 Retinal Macroaneurysm   309
146 Central Retinal Vein Occlusion   311